Nutrition Psychology
Improving Dietary Adherence

MELINDA C. BLACKMAN, PHD
California State University, Fullerton

COLLEEN A. KVASKA, MS, RD
California State University, Fullerton

JONES AND BARTLETT PUBLISHERS
Sudbury, Massachusetts
BOSTON   TORONTO   LONDON   SINGAPORE

World Headquarters

Jones and Bartlett Publishers
40 Tall Pine Drive
Sudbury, MA 01776
978-443-5000
info@jbpub.com
www.jbpub.com

Jones and Bartlett Publishers
Canada
6339 Ormindale Way
Mississauga, Ontario L5V 1J2
Canada

Jones and Bartlett Publishers
International
Barb House, Barb Mews
London W6 7PA
United Kingdom

Jones and Bartlett's books and products are available through most bookstores and online book-sellers. To contact Jones and Bartlett Publishers directly, call 800-832-0034, fax 978-443-8000, or visit our website, www.jbpub.com.

Substantial discounts on bulk quantities of Jones and Bartlett's publications are available to corporations, professional associations, and other qualified organizations. For details and specific discount information, contact the special sales department at Jones and Bartlett via the above contact information or send an email to specialsales@jbpub.com.

The authors, editor, and publisher have made every effort to provide accurate information. However, they are not responsible for errors, omissions, or for any outcomes related to the use of the contents of this book and take no responsibility for the use of the products and procedures described. Treatments and side effects described in this book may not be applicable to all people; likewise, some people may require a dose or experience a side effect that is not described herein. Drugs and medical devices are discussed that may have limited availability controlled by the Food and Drug Administration (FDA) for use only in a research study or clinical trial. Research, clinical practice, and government regulations often change the accepted standard in this field. When consideration is being given to use of any drug in the clinical setting, the health care provider or reader is responsible for determining FDA status of the drug, reading the package insert, and reviewing prescribing information for the most up-to-date recommendations on dose, precautions, and contraindications, and determining the appropriate usage for the product. This is especially important in the case of drugs that are new or seldom used.

Production Credits

Publisher, Higher Education: Cathleen Sether
Acquisitions Editor: Shoshanna Goldberg
Senior Associate Editor: Amy Bloom
Production Director: Amy Rose
Associate Production Editor: Julia Waugaman
Associate Marketing Manager: Jody Sullivan
V. P., Manufacturing and Inventory Control: Therese Connell
Composition: Glyph International
Cover Design: Scott Moden
Photo Research and Permissions Manager: Kimberly Potvin
Associate Photo Researcher: Jessica Elias
Printing and Binding: Malloy Incorporated
Cover Printing: Malloy Incorporated

Library of Congress Cataloging-in-Publication Data
Blackman, Melinda C. (Melinda Carroll)
 Nutrition psychology : improving dietary adherence / Melinda C. Blackman, Colleen A. Kvaska.
   p. ; cm.
 Includes bibliographical references and index.
 ISBN 978-0-7637-8040-1
 1. Diet. 2. Nutrition--Psychological aspects. 3. Food preferences. I. Kvaska, Colleen A. II. Title.
 [DNLM: 1. Diet—psychology. 2. Food Habits—psychology. 3. Food Preferences—psychology. 4. Health Behavior. 5. Health Knowledge, Attitudes, Practice. QT 235 B629n 2011]
 RA784.B5519 2011
 613.2—dc22
                                                                    2010000295

6048

Printed in the United States of America
14 13 12 11 10   10 9 8 7 6 5 4 3 2 1

Contents

Acknowledgments

We are very grateful for the expertise and support of our dedicated editors at J&B, Katey Bircher and Maro Gartside. Thanks for bringing this project to fruition! A special thanks to our agent Stan Wakefield for his hard work and much-appreciated advice along the way. We would also like to thank our reviewers for their time and insight.

M.B. and C.K.

I would like to thank my family for their love and support during this project and encouraging me to follow my dreams. Also, a big thank you goes out to my academic mentor, Dr. David Funder, who is a wonderful role model and made my academic training first rate! Last, I would like to say thank you to my coauthor Colleen. I so enjoyed working on this project with you and am very grateful for all of your knowledge and wisdom.

M.B.

Thank you to Melinda for providing me the opportunity to collaborate and contribute to this unique and insightful textbook.

C.K.

Introduction

For years, the field of psychology has been applied to other disciplines to enhance our quality of life. Psychology has been applied to the field of sports so that athletes can maximize their ability on the playing field and to the legal system so that the validity of eyewitness memory can be better understood. Businesses have long relied on psychologists for selection methods and tests for personnel, yet one discipline has yet to be tapped—the field of nutrition. As obesity and type II diabetes continue to dramatically rise in the United States, the timing for a partnership between the fields of psychology and nutrition (adherence) could not be more opportune. We are excited to bring you this unique partnership between the two disciplines in the form of this textbook.

This text was written with a variety of students and practitioners in mind. We believe that health science, kinesiology, and psychology students; nurses; nutritionists; and doctors, as well as patients, will benefit from the information and practical applications illustrated in this text. The text encompasses all types of dietary adherence programs such as gluten-free, weight-loss, low-sodium, and a nutritionally balanced regimen.

Psychological research has long shown that human behavior can be analyzed and understood from several different perspectives (e.g., behavioral, cognitive, biological, psychoanalytic). We have devoted each chapter in the text to a different psychological perspective while illustrating that perspective's practical applications to nutrition adherence. The reader will become aware of how the environment, a person's cognitions and emotions, one's biology, and even the subconscious all play a role in the extent to which he or she adheres to a prescribed nutrition regimen. After presenting relevant research findings in each chapter, adherence strategies, application illustrations, and workbook-type exercises will be given.

We hope that this text will serve as a springboard for future collaborations between researchers in the fields of psychology and nutrition. May your journey through the text be enlightening!

About the Authors

Dr. Melinda Blackman is a professor of psychology at California State University–Fullerton. Dr. Blackman received her bachelor's degree in psychology from Stanford University and her doctorate in psychology from the University of California–Riverside. Dr. Blackman teaches and conducts research on eating and exercise behavior at the university. She is also the author of *Mind Your Diet: The Psychology Behind Sticking to Any Diet* (2008).

Colleen Kvaska is an adjunct faculty member in the health science department at California State University–Fullerton and an instructor at Fullerton College. She received her bachelor's degree in dietetics from Central Michigan University and her master's degree in family and consumer sciences from California State University–Long Beach. Ms. Kvaska is a registered dietitian and certified diabetes educator. She has worked as a clinical dietitian for over 20 years.

Reviewers

Laurel Branen, PhD, RD, LD
Professor, Food and Nutrition
University of Idaho, Moscow

Cynthia A. Thomson, PhD, RD, FADA
Associate Professor, Nutritional Sciences
University of Arizona, Tucson

Chapter 1

The Discipline of Psychology and Nutrition Adherence: A Logical Partnership

How is it possible that Ronald McDonald is the second most recognizable icon, next to Santa Claus, for this generation's children? More than likely, some extremely clever advertisers on Madison Avenue are responsible for making the public loyal to this food brand. This, of course, is not the only explanation for how nearly 4 million children, ages 6–11, and 5.3 million adolescents, ages 12–19, were overweight or obese in 2002, according to the American Heart Association or that since 1991, the prevalence of obesity among American adults has increased 75 percent.[1,2] However, with the coming of age of eye-catching prepackaged foods, fast food outlets that offer toys and incentives with each meal, super-sized portions, and ever-increasing time demands on our lives, adhering to a healthy eating pattern is becoming more and more difficult. It seems as if these by-products of modern society are thwarting our efforts and clouding our thinking when it comes to eating in our best interest.

As a society, we are very fortunate to have at our disposal a plethora of nutrition and health-based knowledge; however, integrating this knowledge into our demanding lives is becoming increasingly difficult. Now, the time is ripe for the discipline of psychology to provide the bridge between nutritional information and using this information to adhere to a healthy eating pattern. As you will soon see, the relationship between psychology and the field of nutrition is a logical and natural relationship.

A WORD ABOUT PSYCHOLOGY

Before understanding the benefits that the discipline of psychology can have on nutrition adherence, it is important to have a comprehensive grasp of the field of psychology. Many individuals have a limited perspective of the field of psychology. Usually what comes to mind when one hears the word "psychologist" is an image of a therapist analyzing a patient's thoughts. This area of psychology, known as clinical psychology, is only one aspect of what psychologists study. Many psychologists are actually research scientists and use humans as their subjects to test their theories of human nature. The formal definition of psychology from the *Concise Oxford Dictionary* is "the scientific study of the human mind and its functions, especially those affecting behavior in a given context."[3]

Research psychologists study an extremely diverse range of issues such as how humans learn, remember, and process new information. There are psychologists who research the personality characteristics of those individuals with high and low self-esteem and those researchers who study athletes and the mental factors that lead to their peak performances. Psychologists even study the role that genetics play in personality formation from infancy to old age. Of particular importance to this book, there are psychologists who focus their research on eating behavior. As you can see, psychologists study and research the entire gamut of human behavior, both normal and abnormal. Just as medical researchers do, research psychologists use the scientific method (the collection of data through observation or experimentation) to test their hypotheses, frequently with an independent variable (a variable that the experimenter manipulates) and dependent variable (the outcome variable or human behavior) and then publish their findings and theories in professional journals.

GATHERING INFORMATION WITH VARIOUS RESEARCH METHODS

One common thread that ties most research psychologists together is the goal of understanding and predicting human behavior. In particular, psychologists are innately curious as to what propels our behavior in specific and general situations. They might investigate questions such as "Are individuals likely to consume more calories when having a meal by themselves or with other individuals present at the table?" or "Are there specific colors that stimulate an individual's desire to eat?" These research questions can be tested using a variety of research methods that will give us information about how a typical person will behave in a specific situation. Psychologists do not rely entirely on experimental methods to test their hypotheses, but instead examine the research question from various methodological designs.

Experimental Method

Let's look back at the question "Are individuals likely to consume more calories when having a meal by themselves or with other individuals present at the table?" A researcher could test this question and implement any one of at least seven different research methods. By testing this question with an experimental design, the researcher would form two conditions: a control condition in which the participant eats their meal alone and the experimental condition in which the participant is surrounded with two or three acquaintances at his or her table. The independent variable in the study would be the number of people present at the dining table, while the dependent variable would be operationalized as the number of calories consumed by the participant.

Observational (Obtrusive Versus Unobtrusive) Method

This same research question could be tested using an observational research method approach as well. An observational design involves observing and recording human behavior in a natural environment. Two types of observational designs exist: the obtrusive design and the unobtrusive design. Participants in obtrusive designs are informed that their behavior is being viewed or monitored, whereas those participants in an unobtrusive design are unaware that their behavior is being recorded or observed. As you can imagine there are advantages and disadvantages to both designs. With an obtrusive design, the participant knows that he or she is being observed and may feel obligated to change his or her behavior so that it is a socially desirable behavior. This action possibly confirms the researcher's hypothesis. However, participants in an unobtrusive design are unaware that they are in a study and will probably give the researcher a true glimpse of their unstaged behavior. (A prominent disadvantage of the unobtrusive approach though is the ethical issue of recording an individual's behavior without their consent.)

A researcher who wants to use the unobtrusive observational approach to study the previous research question might use a fast food restaurant, where the calorie count of each menu item is printed on the wrapper. With this knowledge, the researcher would position him- or herself in the restaurant for a 2-hour period and observe all patrons who are dining alone in the restaurant. For each patron, the researcher would record the items that he or she had on their tray and whether that person ate all items. Then, the next day during the same time period, that researcher would observe all individuals who had one or more individuals dining with them at their table. Again the researcher would record the items on the target participant's tray and whether he or she ate all of the meal items. Ideally, the mean number of calories consumed by individuals dining alone would be significantly less than the number of calories consumed by patrons dining with one or more individuals.

Food Record Data

This same research question can be investigated using food records. This retrospective method involves asking the research participants to record their eating behavior at a certain point during the day. Usually the researcher provides the participants with a journal or a food log for each day of the week with preprinted questions to be answered (e.g., how many individuals were present at the table for breakfast, for lunch, for dinner?). The researcher would also have the participant record what they ate at each meal as well as the quantity. One disadvantage to food record data is that it is retrospective and this type of data can be subject to several memory errors on the part of the participant, such as forgetting, bias recall, and socially desirable responding. Research indicates that participants completing food records underreport their actual food intake by 27 to 46 percent.[4] However, in defense of using food records, research also indicates that participants lose more weight when food records are kept. In addition, the researcher would be obtaining real life and daily information from the participant, whereas, in an experimental study, the situation is artificially contrived; the results of the study would have lower generalizability to daily life situations and behavior.

Experience Sampling

A newer research method that can be used to test research questions is the experience sampling method. This method involves alerting participants at variable intervals during the day to stop their current behavior and record it immediately on a printed template that the researcher has provided. Typically, the participants are given pagers to wear and are beeped at various intervals throughout the day (sometimes up to a half a dozen times). The participants are unaware of when they will be beeped during the day and are asked to carry on with their daily life as usual. Experience sample studies can last from 1 day to a month or more. Experience sampling is one of the optimal ways psychologists have of obtaining a participant's natural minute-to-minute behavior. One disadvantage to this technique is that some participants have been known to experience "beeper anxiety" and stop all daily activities in anticipation of the beeper going off, much to the researcher's dismay.

Survey Data (Self Report Versus Peer Data)

One of the most common (and sometimes overused) research methods that psychologists implement is the survey method. Surveys can typically consist of open-ended questions (e.g., Write down everything you ate for breakfast), fixed option questions (e.g., How many calories did you consume for breakfast? A. 0–100; B. 101–200; C. 201–300, etc.) or food frequency checklists (e.g., Place a checkmark next to each food item on the list that you consumed during your last meal).

Survey data is usually completed by the participant and this is known as self data. As one can surmise, there are advantages and disadvantages to having the target participant complete a survey. One advantage to having the participant complete a survey is the participant knows themselves better than anyone else. The participant is indeed the best expert regarding themselves and their personal experiences with their own eating behaviors. However, as mentioned earlier, participants are sometimes subject to forgetting information and of course embellishing information in order to look more socially acceptable to the researcher.

Due to these factors, many researchers are now asking a well-acquainted friend, peer, or family member to complete surveys about the participant; this type of data is known as informant data.[5] By having not only the participant's perspective about their eating behavior, but that of a good acquaintance as well, a clearer picture of the target participant's behavior will hopefully come into view for the researcher. However, just as self data can be tainted by various factors, so too can informant data. Friends and family members may not have experienced every situation with the target participant or they could bring bias recall into the survey data as well. For these reasons, it is important when gathering survey data to use an increasingly popular method that industrial/organizational psychologists (psychologist who study human behavior in the workplace) use: 360-degree feedback.[6] When these psychologists evaluate employees' performance in the workplace, they typically gather survey data about the employee's performance from everyone who interacts with the employee on a daily or weekly basis (e.g., customers, coworkers, a supervisor, and the employee's subordinates) as well as the employee themselves. Each perspective gives the researcher another piece of the target participant's overall behavior in various situations. These perspectives are sometimes averaged to give the participant an overall performance evaluation score. Three hundred and sixty degree feedback is also very applicable to the field of nutrition. This method will allow the researcher to gather more information about the target subject's eating behavior that he or she may not be even aware of, but can be clearly seen from the vantage point of a peer or family member. The more perspectives that a researcher can obtain about a target participant's behavior; the more likely she or he will accrue valid and reliable data.

Multiple Method Approach

With numerous methods to choose from to test research questions, one is left to wonder which approach is the best. There is clearly no one methodological approach that is superior to the others. However, what is advocated in the field of psychology is to examine research questions from multiple approaches and to utilize multiple methods.[7] If the results from an experimental study, a survey study, and a food record data study all confirm that indeed people are more likely to consume more calories at a meal when other diners are present at the table, researchers can feel more confident that this phenomenon is a robust occurrence and the results can be extrapolated to other populations of individuals in a variety of eating contexts. However, if this finding was confirmed through only a series of experimental studies, the generalizability of the phenomenon occurring outside of the laboratory would be tenuous at best. Ultimately, utilizing multiple research methods to test a research question will give a more complete and truthful picture of human nature than will the reliance on one methodological approach.

THEORETICAL PERSPECTIVES

Through the years, several major theoretical perspectives have been developed to account for the factors that drive human behavior. Some of the most prominent theoretical perspectives include cognitive, biological, behavioral, evolutionary, psychoanalytic, humanistic, and the trait theory. We will give an overview of each of these perspectives, because the strategies on nutrition adherence given in the upcoming chapters will be based upon combinations of these psychological perspectives.

The Cognitive Perspective

Psychologists who adopt the cognitive perspective believe or research the role that our cognitions (thoughts), perceptions, emotions, and motivation processes fuel our behavior. To illustrate this perspective, suppose a psychologist wanted to investigate the reason behind the finding that hot colors such as red, orange, and bright yellow are known to stimulate human mood and appetite.[8] As cognitive psychologists, they would start by examining participants' thoughts and perceptions when shown various colors. They might also explore participants' differences in *priming*. Priming refers to concepts that have been recently activated or cued by something that happened today and are quick to come to mind with even only a little stimulus.[9] Participants who have just watched a food-related commercial on television or passed by the vibrant colors of a McDonald's or Burger King restaurant are considered *primed* to eat; when shown a bright vibrant color, this might stimulate feelings of hunger.

Emotions are another cognitive process that can be examined with regard to stimulating appetite. *Emotions* can be defined as a set of mental and physical procedures that one learns through inner experiences. For some individuals, emotional change can be a stimulus for appetite; in other individuals, a particular eating pattern may elicit positive reinforcing emotions. For example, a working mother may come home after an 8-hour work day, cook dinner for her family, help her children with homework, throw a load of clothes in the washer, prepare her children's lunches for the next day, and put her children to bed. When she finally has time to relax, she gets a bowl of ice cream and sits down in front of the TV. Eating the ice cream initiates positive pleasurable emotions and helps her to relax. Therefore, she may begin to develop a pattern of eating ice cream every night after her children are in bed in order to stimulate those same emotions. Conversely, emotions can serve either as antecedents to eating behavior or as by-products of such behavior.

Cognitive psychologists are also fascinated by how much of human behavior can be attributed to an individual's constant efforts to achieve his or her goals. Whether a goal is short term or long term, an individual's life is characterized by what Eric Klinger (1981) calls current concerns.[10] A *current concern* is an ongoing motivation that persists in one's mind until the goal is either attained or the goal is abandoned. Many current concerns can bring arousing emotions to mind as well. Suppose an individual had the long-term goal of drinking eight 8 oz. glasses of water a day. This individual's current concern during each day would likely be "Have I been keeping up with my intended water intake?" If, during the course of the day, he perceives he is not on the path to attaining his goal, then certain emotions will be aroused (e.g., frustration, anxiety). As you can see, many of our cognitive processes naturally interact with one another and ultimately preempt our behavior, or relevant to this text, our eating behavior.

The Biological Perspective

Researchers who advocate the biological perspective delve into the theory that our brain anatomy, neurophysiology, and genes influence our behavior. Thanks to modern technology (e.g., EEG machines, PET scanners and MRI scans) we are able to examine the brain's anatomy to understand its relationship to the brain and our behavior. Through technology, it has been discovered that just about every structure of the brain is related to our personality in some way. However, the interactions between various structures of the brain and its effects on our mind and behavior are just beginning to be studied and understood.

Another area that biopsychologists, psychologists who analyze how the brain and its neurotransmitters influence our behaviors, are concerned with is the extent to which our biochemistry (e.g., neurotransmitters and hormones) is responsible for our personalities and behavior, particularly eating behavior. Studies from the University of Minnesota–St. Paul and the University of British Columbia–Vancouver provide relevant examples of the relationship between our biochemistry and our eating patterns. Researchers from these universities have confirmed that women get hungrier during the 2 weeks following ovulation (usually days 14 to 28 of the menstrual cycle).[11] That is when the body's metabolic rate climbs, most likely in response to an increased secretion of the hormone progesterone, which causes the body to burn calories at a faster rate and in turn intensifies appetite.

Researchers are also discovering hormones and neurotransmitters produced by fat cells and the gastrointestinal tract. They believe these hormones and neurotransmitters act upon the hypothalamus and communicate with the brain influencing satiety and appetite. For example, the hormone leptin is manufactured in fat cells and in the stomach.[12] It signals the brain that the body has a sufficient storage of energy (fat) and suppresses appetite. Leptin is also manufactured by cells in the stomach when food is consumed and affects levels of satiety. Researchers believe that some individuals, due to their physiological or genetic makeup, may not produce leptin at all, produce it in an insufficient amount, or produce too much but have a resistance to it. These individuals, therefore, have difficulty recognizing feelings of satiety, consume more calories than their body requires, and develop obesity. Another hormone, ghrelin, is manufactured by cells in the stomach.[13] It stimulates appetite and promotes body fat storage. This hormone also plays a role in sleep regulation. A person who gets an insufficient amount of sleep will manufacture more ghrelin which in turn stimulates appetite. It is theorized that some people may genetically or biochemically be inclined to produce more or less of these hormones that affect appetite stimulation and satiety signals and ultimately, regulation of body weight.[14]

It is also important to note that our environments can affect the bio-chemistry in our bodies. Individuals who are facing serious environmental stressors induce their bodies into a state of flight or fight. In this state, the body typically responds by cutting off the digestive process in order to conserve energy and thus decreasing one's desire to eat. On the other hand, chronic stress caused by work, low socioeconomic status, and depression are associated with an increased risk of obesity, particularly in women.[15] Obesity is associated with inflammation and it is found that obese humans have increased blood levels of various cytokines, blood markers of inflammation, during times of stress. Researchers are just beginning to understand the interactions between environmental triggers and human biochemistry and the effect that they have on eating behaviors.

The Behavioral Perspective

Behavioral psychologists view human behavior as stemming from the rewards and punishments from our past or current environments.[16] The philosophical roots of behaviorism are planted in empiricism, which is the belief that all knowledge comes from experience and also that of associationism, which is the idea that paired stimuli will come to be regarded as one. So, from these philosophical roots, we can see the logic that behaviorism is also referred to as the learning perspective. Learning is termed as any change in behavior that results from experience. The behaviorist perspective embraces several basic principles of learning including habituation, classical conditioning, operant conditioning, and social learning, which will be discussed in greater detail in upcoming chapters.

If a behaviorist was to account for how certain colors were responsible for stimulating our appetites, she would likely look back at our past experiences with color. She might be able to trace an individual whose appetite is stimulated each time he sees the color yellow to the fact that when growing up, this person's kitchen and dining room were predominantly furnished in hues of yellow. Through countless mealtime pairings of food being prepared and eaten in a yellow environment, this individual would have learned that the color yellow signals that food is present or is about to be ingested. His body, after these many learning trials, has learned that the color yellow signals food and his body then reacts by stimulating the appetite. Many times much of our learning takes place under our conscious radar and it is only after retracing our past experiences and environments can we piece together how that behavior was learned and its origins.

The Evolutionary Perspective

The evolutionary perspective is an extension of the theorizing that began with Charles Darwin's *Origin of Species* (1859).[17] Darwin's theories and book compared one species of animal or plant to another to explain the functional significance of various aspects of anatomy and behavior. Recently, psychologists have been extrapolating this same kind of theorizing and reasoning to human behavior. The evolutionary perspective assumes that behaviors seen in people today are present because these behaviors were necessary for survival. In other words, the more a behavior helps an individual to survive or reproduce, the more likely the behavior is to occur in future generations.

An evolutionary psychologist who wanted to understand human eating behavior might look at the survival significance of various eating patterns. For instance, this psychologist might note the tendency for humans to consume more calories during the fall/harvest months when compared to the spring and summer months.[18] The psychologist, in keeping with the evolutionary perspective, would probably view this tendency as crucial to human survival, in that it allowed humans to store up fat for the winter months when food was scarce. Turning back to our original question concerning the ability of colors to stimulate human appetite, an evolutionary psychologist would again look for the survival function that carefully discerning color produces. She might focus on how nature signifies healthy fruits for us to eat through the use of vibrant colors (e.g., ripe red apples, bright yellow bananas) and how these vibrant colors through time have come to stimulate human appetite. Conversely, nature through the use of color alerts us to which foods are dangerous and we should not eat (e.g., green mold, odd spots, less vibrant colors). Evolutionary psychologists would argue that various eating patterns, though not adaptive presently, were adaptive for human survival at some point in history.

The Psychoanalytic Perspective

The psychoanalytic perspective was developed by Sigmund Freud and posits that most aspects of our mental life (e.g., thoughts, feelings, motives, and the resulting behavior) are unconscious, which is why we have a difficult time understanding our own behavior.[19] Freud theorized that forbidden impulses and desires in our unconscious mind are responsible for our everyday behavior. He believed that many of these impulses were developed during stages that we passed through in early childhood and it is only after getting in touch with the unconscious portion of the mind can one uncover the roots of their behavior. Freud used techniques such as hypnosis and free association with words to uncover some of the impulses and desires stirring under the conscious radar. By bringing these impulses and desires to the surface, one can resolve these maladaptive behaviors.

Freud also focused much of his studies on the topic of internal and external anxiety. Freud coined the term *psychic conflict* as a state of anxiety when our mind is battling itself; in other words, when our desires are battling our morals of what is right and wrong. Freud discussed a variety of tools that our minds use to keep our anxiety levels within a tolerable range, whether the anxiety was internally generated or from stressors of the external world. One of the simplest defense mechanism is denial—where one simply refuses to acknowledge the source of anxiety. Rationalization is another defense mechanism that we use to keep stress a bay. If we have undertaken some sort of shameless behavior, we concoct a seemingly rational case for why we had to undertake that behavior. A psychoanalytic psychologist, who was examining dysfunctional eating behavior, would likely try to uncover the source of anxiety, while looking at the defense mechanisms used to cope with it. We will discuss these defense mechanisms in detail in upcoming chapters and their interplay with eating behavior.

Freud had many protégés who built on his ideas relating to the roots of human behavior. One in particular, Mary Ainsworth, put forth the idea that much of our behavior is due to how we were attached at birth to 2 years of age to our primary caregiver, typically our mother.[20] Ainsworth believed that our attachment style predicted much of our future behavior in life. Children who developed what Ainsworth calls a "secure attachment style" to their mothers and felt comfortable that she would meet their needs, would display well-adjusted behavior throughout life, confident faith in themselves, and form secure attachments with their future romantic partners. However, children who had an "anxious-ambivalent attachment style" to their mothers, and felt that she was not always there to meet their needs, would potentially display neurotic behavior and have dysfunctional future relationships with others. Children who formed "avoidant" relationships with their caregivers, usually came from homes where they had been rebuffed in their attempts to enjoy contact with their primary caregiver. These individuals, Ainsworth believed, would have a hard time in life coping with stress and would be more likely to deny that it exists. Psychologists who foster this perspective of human behavior examine eating behavior as a byproduct of the attachment style that the target individual developed with their primary caregiver. The psychoanalytic perspective is a complex interplay of unconscious components, yet much of it revolves around the issue of tension and anxiety.

The Humanistic Perspective

Another way of accounting for the forces that drive human behavior is the humanistic perspective. Advocates of this theory believe that every human being is uniquely different in the experiences that they have encountered throughout life.[21] Through these experiences, each person develops their own constructs or lens through which they interpret their surroundings; this lens is ultimately responsible for their behavior. Humanistic psychologists focus in on our unique experience of the world called our *construal*. Construals are interpretations rather than direct reflections of reality; they can be freely chosen and different from anyone else's. Humanistic psychologists strongly believe that only after you have "walked in another person's shoes" or experienced their unique view of reality can you begin to understand what drives their behavior. More specifically, if one were to utilize the same constructs and perspective on life as the target participant, then one could develop an understanding of the forces that are driving that individual's behavior.

When working to find the types of lens that the target participant views the world through, humanistic psychologists use a technique termed unconditional positive regard. *Unconditional positive regard* is giving respect and affirmation to the target participant regardless of what they believe or say as they are revealing their own construct system and the lens through which they process the world. Carl Rogers and Abraham Maslow, two humanistic psychologists who began their research in the 1950s, believe that a person's ultimate need or motive in life is to self-actualize, which is to maintain and enhance life. Maslow, however, believed that before one could begin to self-actualize, they need to have their basic needs met (e.g., food, water, safety, a sense of belonging, and esteem).[22] Rogers and Maslow advocated that the optimal way to live is to accurately perceive the world without neurotic distortion: If you take responsibility for the choices that you make, you will become a fully functioning person. A fully functioning person faces the world without fear, self-doubt, and neurotic defenses. The only way to develop into this type of individual is to receive unconditional positive regard and affirmation from the important people in your life, such as your parents, relatives, and friends.

A humanistic psychologist researching eating behavior would examine two important aspects of an individual's life: "Have their basic needs been met?" and "Have they received unconditional positive regard and affirmation from those they value?" If the answer is "no" to these two questions, then meeting the individual's basic needs and making sure those around him provide unconditional positive regard would be a humanistic psychologist's prescription for any type of abnormal eating behavior, because these aspects are obstructing the individual from becoming fully functional.

The Trait Perspective

The last perspective that will be incorporated in this text is the trait perspective. Trait psychologists believe that individuals differ in their characteristic patterns of thought, feeling, and behavior; these patterns are called personality traits. In fact, personality traits are such an important part of life, Allport and his graduate student Odbert (1936) researched the dictionary and complied a list of 17,953 words in the English language that describe an individual's personality.[23] Trait psychologists hold the belief that individual behavior is the result of each person's unique and dynamic traits. Many trait proponents generally believe that biological influences, such as genes and prenatal hormones, produce children with particular childhood temperaments; some children are active and aggressive, while others are quieter. However, it is through life experiences that these temperament styles are molded into individual stable traits (e.g., is outgoing, is shy). The ultimate goal of trait psychologists is to predict future human behavior accurately and to increase our understanding of the reasons for human behavior.

A Perspective Controversy

No one perspective can account for all types of human behavior 100 percent of the time, but it is important to be open to the idea that these perspectives interact with one another to account for and predict human behavior. This idea that theoretical perspectives can interact with one another was a rather novel idea about 40 years in the history of the field.

In 1968, a prominent psychologist at Stanford University named Walter Mischel published a controversial book entitled *Personality and Assessment*.[24] In his book, Mischel argued that human behavior is extremely inconsistent from one situation to another; because of that, researchers cannot accurately assess an individual with personality traits. There was a prominent debate between research psychologists concerning what causes a person's behavior. Some researchers firmly believed that human behavior is solely based upon personality-related thoughts, while other researchers upheld that the situation a person finds him- or herself in causes their behavior. The researchers argued for about 20 years on this subject (later titled *The Person-Situation Debate*). Based on the results of several studies, they came to one conclusion: A person's behavior in a particular situation is best predicted by an interaction or combination of the person's traits and the situational circumstances.[25] Similarly, psychologists who study human eating behavior have also concluded that individual and environmental factors interact together to influence eating behaviors.

THE LAYOUT OF THE TEXTBOOK

During the course of this textbook, we will closely examine these psychological perspectives that are believed to drive human (eating) behavior. Within each chapter, you will become acquainted with research findings that illustrate the basis for eating patterns relevant to that particular psychological perspective. The latter half of each chapter will consist of tangible illustrations of psychological strategies known to counteract dysfunctional eating patterns so one can adhere to healthy and/or prescribed eating patterns.

As stated earlier, it is fortunate that today we have a plethora of knowledge about human dietary needs and imbalances. This information can live up to its lifesaving potential when coupled with the field of psychology because the time is ripe for a merger between nutrition and psychology. The field of psychology provides a logical lens through which to understand human eating patterns and an optimal vehicle to disseminate strategies of nutrition adherence.

REFERENCES

1. American Heart Association. (2004). *End of the Year Report.* Dallas, TX: American Heart Association News.
2. Blackman, M. (2008). Mind Your Diet: The Psychology Behind Sticking to Any Diet. Xlibris Corporation.
3. Soanes, C., & Stevenson, A. (Eds.). (2008). *Concise Oxford Dictionary.* Oxford, England: Oxford University Press.
4. Paul, D.R., Rhodes, D.G., Kramer, M., Baer, D.J., & Rumpler, W.V. (2005). Validation of a food frequency questionnaire by direct measurement of habitual ad libitum food intake. *American Journal of Epidemiology, 162*(8), 806–814.
5. Funder, D.C., & Colvin, C.R. (1991). Explorations in behavioral consistency: Properties of persons, situations, and behaviors. *Journal of Personality and Social Psychology, 60,* 773–794.
6. Atkins, P., & Wood, R. (2002). Self-versus others' ratings as predictors of assessment center ratings: Validation evidence for 360-degree feedback programs. *Personnel Psychology, 55*(4), 871–904.
7. Campbell, D.T., & Fiske, D.W. (1959). Convergent and discriminant validation by the multitrait-multimethod matrix. *Psychological Bulletin, 56,* 81–105.
8. Wansink, B. (2006). *Mindless Eating—Why We Eat More Than We Think.* New York: Bantam-Dell.

9. Neely, J.H. (1977). Semantic priming and retrieval from lexical memory: Roles of inhibitionless spreading activation and limited-capacity attention. *Journal of Experimental Psychology: General, 106,* 226–254.

10. Klinger, E., Barta, S.G., & Maxeiner, M.E. (1981). Current concerns: Assessing therapeutically relevant motivation. In P.C. Kendall & S. Hollon (Eds.), *Assessment Strategies for Cognitive-Behavioral Interventions* (pp. 161–195). New York: Academic.

11. Michener, W. (1999). The role of low progesterone and tension as triggers of perimenstrual chocolate and sweets craving: Some negative experimental evidence. *Physiology and Behavior, 67,* 417–420.

12. Keim, N., Stern, J., & Havel, P. (1998). Relation between circulating leptin concentrations and appetite during a prolonged, moderate energy deficit in women. *American Journal of Clinical Nutrition, 68*(4), 794–801.

13. Cummings, D., Weigle, D., Frayo, R., Breen, P., Ma, M., Dellinger, E., et al. (2002). Plasma ghrelin levels after diet-induced weight loss or gastric bypass surgery. *New England Journal of Medicine, 34*(21), 1623–1630.

14. Weigle, D.S., Cummings, D.E., Newby, P.D., Breen, P.A., Frayo, R.S., Matthy, C.C., et al. (2003). Roles of leptin and ghrelin in the loss of body weight caused by a low fat, high carbohydrate diet. *Journal of Clinical Endocrinology & Metabolism, 88*(4), 1577–1586.

15. Adam, T.C., & Epel, E.S. (2007). Stress, eating and the reward system. *Physiological Behavior, 91*(4), 449–458.

16. Watson, J.B. (1912). Psychology as the behaviorist views it. *Psychological Review, 20,* 158–177.

17. Darwin, C. (1859). *On the Origin of Species by Means of Natural Selection, or the Preservation of Favoured Races in the Struggle for Life* (1st ed.). John Murray: London, England.

18. Ma, Y., Olendzki, B.C., Hafner, A.R., Chiriboga, D., Hebert, J.R., Campbell, M., et al. (2005). Seasonal variation in food intake, physical activity, and body weight in a predominantly overweight population. *European Journal of Clinical Nutrition, 60,* 519–528.

19. Freud, A. (1936). *The Ego and the Mechanisms of Defense.* New York: Hogarth.

20. Ainsworth, M.D.S., Blehar, M.C., Waters, E., & Wall, S. (1978). *Patterns of Attachment: Assessed in the Strange Situation and at Home.* Hillsdale, NJ: Erlbaum.

21. Rogers, C. (1961). *On Becoming a Person.* Boston: Houghton Mifflin.

22. Maslow, A.H. (1987). *Motivation and Personality* (3rd ed.). Harper: New York.

23. Allport, G.W., & Odbert, H.S. (1936). Trait-names: A psycho-lexical study. *Psychological Monographs: General and Applied, 47,* 171–220.

24. Mischel, W. (1968). *Personality and Assessment.* New York: Wiley.

25. Kenrick, D.T., & Funder, D.C. (1988). Profiting from controversy: Lessons from the person-situation debate. *American Psychologist, 43,* 23–34.

THE BEHAVIORAL PERSPECTIVE

Chapter 2

Basic Forms of Learning from Our Environment

By the end of this chapter, the reader will be able to:

1. Understand that much of our eating behavior is learned from interactions with our environment.
2. Identify and distinguish between the three forms of basic learning/conditioning in nutrition adherence.
3. Effectively implement a reinforcement system for nutrition adherence.
4. Apply each of the learning theories as strategies to a nutrition-adherence program.

You Keep a Stiff Upper Lip . . .

When your physician gravely gives you the news that your blood pressure is dangerously high. You feel as if a blow has been just delivered when she tells you that she will be putting you on an antihypertensive drug. The doctor reiterates that untreated hypertension can lead to heart failure, a possible stroke, or kidney damage. With those visual images in mind, you consent to taking the daily drug.

After taking the medication for a short period of time, your blood pressure returns to an acceptable level and you sigh with relief. You are silently thankful that you did not need to change your eating habits or give up your highly demanding career to restore your body's balance. You continue to faithfully take the medication daily, as your blood pressure remains at a normal level.

What you are unaware of is that after 3 weeks of being on the medication, your physician replaced your antihypertensive drug with a placebo, a pill that has no actual physiological effect on your body—yet, your body still continued to maintain a normal blood pressure level.

This scenario reflects a finding that Robert Ader and Anthony Suchman found in a series of experiments in which patients who were taken off their hypertensive blood pressure medication and treated with placebos were able to maintain normal blood pressure levels longer than patients who did not get placebos.[1,2]

How can an inert pill cure hypertension? After repeated exposures to the real drug, the physical ritual involved in taking the drug became associated with the physiological changes involved in lowering blood pressure. Patients did not have to learn consciously that a medication reduced the force of their heartbeat, increased salts, and water excreted in the urine. Instead, through repeated association of these effects with the act of taking the medicine, subjects' bodies became conditioned to respond appropriately, even after the active ingredients were withdrawn.

BEHAVIORISM AND ITS PHILOSOPHICAL ROOTS

The previous scenario exemplifies the concept of learning: a change of behavior as a function of experience, and even more specifically, classical conditioning (a form of learning discussed later). There are several ways from which we learn. For example, any time two stimuli (e.g., events, people, or things) are repeatedly experienced at the same time, they will both come to elicit the same response from an individual. Imagine the ringing of a bell and having a jellybean put inside your mouth at the same time. Eventually you will learn to salivate when either hearing the bell or having the jellybean in your mouth.

Another prominent form of learning occurs when a behavior is repeatedly followed by a pleasant outcome. This behavior will tend to be repeated more often while behaviors followed by unpleasant outcomes will be stopped. If a woman feels energized after riding an exercise bike for 20 minutes, then she will continue to engage in this behavior in the future. However, if she feels bloated and experiences digestive problems each time she consumes food with the additive MSG, she will discontinue eating foods with this additive in it. As you can see from both of these forms of learning, our behavior changes as a result of experience. Though psychology is the study of our psyche and what is going on in our heads, researchers who take on the behaviorist perspective believe that the only way to know someone is to watch what he or she does; in other words, their behavior. The roots of the behaviorist perspective come from three philosophical ideas. One of the philosophical ideas comes from empiricism: the idea that all knowledge comes from experience. John Locke, the nineteenth-century philosopher, believed that at birth our minds are a blank slate, a "tabula rasa" and that only experience writes on them.[3] In addition, John Watson, the twentieth-century psychologist and founder of behaviorism, believed that when a person encounters reality and accrues experiences, then he or she builds a characteristic way of reacting to the world.[3]

Associationism is another prominent philosophical idea that attempts to explain how learning occurs. As mentioned earlier, any two events, people, or objects that are repeatedly experienced together become mentally considered as one and, thus, the person's reaction to one also becomes his or her reaction to the other as well.

The last philosophical concept that makes up the behavioral perspective is hedonism, otherwise referred to as motivation. With regard to behaviorism, hedonism advocates that people learn for two purposes: to seek pleasure and to avoid pain. These two basic motivations account for why rewards and punishment form behavior, because people are more likely to consume sweet substances when the reward is positive, than sour/unpalatable or spoiled foods with the negative repercussions of unpleasant aftertastes.

THREE FORMS OF LEARNING

In this chapter, we will discuss three kinds of learning that the behaviorist tradition identifies as being responsible for propelling human behavior: habituation, classical conditioning, and operant conditioning.

Habituation

The simplest form of learning is termed habituation. This form of learning can take place among all living beings, even amoebas. Simply stated, after repeated exposure to the same stimuli, one habituates to it and over time stops responding to the stimuli. For instance, the first bite of a chocolate chip cookie may cause your mouth to salivate and your taste buds to enthusiastically come alive. However, after several bites, your mouth begins to habituate to the sugary stimuli and stops responding with such zest. Eventually, your taste buds stop responding at all, though many of us continue to eat, hoping to regain that original taste explosion in our mouths.

Research on the topic of habituation reveals that in order to obtain a response that is almost as strong as the original response, one would need to change the stimulus slightly or increase the quantity of the original stimulus with each repeated exposure.[4] In other words, if we were to change to a different flavor of cookie or if we increased the quantity of the cookie that we put in our mouth, we would be able to maintain that original taste explosion or be able to maintain that taste sensation for a little while longer. Habituation can occur with personal events as well. Research has shown that lottery winners on the day they win millions of dollars have a tremendous surge in their level of happiness; however, over time, their level of happiness habituates or returns back to its original prelottery level.[5] Dieting behavior also follows this principle. If an overweight individual decides to go to on a diet to lose weight and this is his very first attempt, he usually is quite motivated to follow his food plan. He loses weight by adhering closely to the food plan; however, over time, the food plan becomes more difficult to follow. Several weeks or months later, he finds that his food choices and eating behaviors return back to what they were before he began the diet. This usually results in gaining back the weight he lost and sets him up to anticipate the next "miracle diet" that he is sure will work better for him than the first diet.

Classical Conditioning

The second form of learning that can occur was illustrated in the opening scenario with the body learning that ingesting a specific pill leads to a reduction in one's blood pressure level. From this scenario, we can see that classical conditioning/learning can affect our physiological responses, our emotional responses, and low-level behavioral responses. The concept of classical conditioning was discovered accidentally in the early 1900s by Russian scientist Ivan Pavlov who was originally studying the physiology of digestion and using dogs as his subjects. What turned out to be an unwanted complication in his study resulted in Pavlov winning the Nobel Prize for his work in 1904.[6] Originally, Pavlov was examining how dogs salivate when eating; however, he noticed that they began to salivate before they were fed upon seeing or even hearing the sound of the footsteps of the research assistant who was to feed them. Intrigued with this phenomenon, Pavlov turned to psychology to investigate its cause. Pavlov learned that objects other than food could elicit salivation in the dogs. Through several trials of simultaneously ringing a bell at the time of feeding, Pavlov found that he could induce the dogs to salivate merely upon ringing the bell, even without the presence of food. Ultimately, what Pavlov showed was that conditioning/learning involves teaching an individual that one stimulus can signal the occurrence of another stimulus that is soon to follow. The dogs soon learned to respond to the signaling stimulus (the footsteps of the research assistant) before the actual eliciting stimuli (food) was present.

Eventually the signaling stimulus can be present and elicit a response (salvation) without even encountering the eliciting stimuli (food).

Classical conditioning can also work in the opposite direction. For instance, suppose you ate a spoiled sandwich and became violently ill immediately afterward. The prominent taste that you had while eating the sandwich was parsley. From that point on you develop a strong aversion to the smell and taste of parsley, even though you know that the contributing factor to your illness was the spoiled turkey in the sandwich. Similarly, this example illustrates that concepts become associated not merely because they occurred simultaneously, but because the meaning of one concept has changed the meaning of another. With regard to this example, parsley will be the signal that an upset stomach is going to occur. This example and the opening high blood pressure scenario are tangible examples of unintentional classical conditioning. Unintentional classical conditioning as seen in the opening scenario can change the effects of drugs.

Learned Helplessness

Another form of learning that can affect an individual's future behavior is called learned helplessness in which the person learns that one stimulus is not related to another. This form of learning focuses on the unpredictability of the stimuli and the consequential rewards or punishments. Learned helplessness is best illustrated by experiments with humans who receive electric shocks regardless of what type of behavior they exhibit. This typically leads to the belief that there is no behavior that will stop the shocks from coming and the person gives up responding.[7]

A client on a strict low-sodium eating plan to lower their blood pressure level may find that their blood pressure is not lowered when they adhere to the plan. They also determine that even when they do not follow the low-sodium eating plan their blood pressure is not adversely affected. After several instances of seeing no positive effects of adhering to the low-sodium eating plan, the client will develop the belief that "nothing I do will lower my blood pressure level, so why bother changing my behavior." With this evidence-based belief, the patient may decide to stop trying to adhere to any type of proactive behavior, including the low-sodium eating plan, to lower their blood pressure.

Operant Conditioning

A frequently used type of learning that will be discussed in this chapter is referred to as operant conditioning and was studied by the American psychologist Edward Thorndike in the early 1900s. Like Pavlov, Thorndike used animals as his test subjects—hungry cats in Thorndike's case. Thorndike put the hungry cat in a box called a puzzle box. The cats could only escape the box by pulling on a wire or pressing a bar. Upon exhibiting this specific behavior, the puzzle box would spring open and the cat would jump out to find a piece of food within close proximity. After several trials, Thorndike found that the cats were catching on to the puzzle box and were escaping quicker and quicker with each trial.[8] Through trial and error, the cats had gained insight and learned the specific behavior that it took to receive the reward when released from the box.

Later, a psychologist working in this area, B.F. Skinner coined this form of learning operant conditioning, alluding to the fact that the animals had learned to manipulate their own world in order to be rewarded for that behavior. Skinner developed a box similar to Thorndike's puzzle box and named it the Skinner Box.[9] Skinner typically put pigeons or rats inside the Skinner Box. Inside the box, the pigeon in the course of moving around would randomly push a bar and a food pellet would fall down the shoot. The pigeon would then eat it and then go about exploring the box, unintentionally pushing the bar again. The food pellet would again drop down the shoot and the pigeon would eat it. Eventually, the pigeon would catch on and learned how to control his environment in the Skinner Box in order to obtain as much food as he wanted. Skinner found that the pigeons would keep up this behavior as long as they were positively reinforced by food. Conversely, this behavior would be stopped or extinguished if it was followed by a punishment such as a spurt of cold water falling down the shoot.

Operant conditioning can also shape or modify an individual's behavior so that it becomes more complex. This process of eliciting more difficult behavior from the subject can be done through gradual steps that increase the criterion for a reward. The pigeon that originally received a food pellet after pushing the bar may determine that it has to not only press the bar but also pull a wire with its beak for the food pellet to be dispersed. Through trial and error, the pigeon will learn that the criterion has been raised in order to receive reinforcement. This molding of more complex behavior is referred to as shaping.

APPLICABLE STRATEGIES FOR NUTRITION ADHERENCE

Strategies to Counteract Habitual Eating Behavior

In the second part of this chapter, nutrition adherence strategies will be given with regard to each form of learning. Remember that habituation is the most basic form of learning and can occur without conscious awareness;

habituation research has been conducted with regard to human and animal eating patterns. The habituation theory applied to eating would suggest that repeated exposure to food stimuli would result in a decreased response to the sensory properties of the food and potentially provide a sense of satiation for the food.[10,11] In addition, the habituation theory would also suggest that the rate of habituation is dependent on the intensity of the stimulus (food). For example, one would be quicker to habituate to bland-tasting foods than foods that have a variety of different flavors. Similarly, if one consumes a large quantity of a specific food in one mouthful, this, too, will act as an intense stimulus. Especially for foods that one likes, there is a natural tendency for people, when they start to experience habituation to the food, to proportionally increase the quantity of that food in each mouthful, creating a false sense of stimuli intensity. This false sense of stimuli intensity staves off a sense of satiety while promoting overeating. This type of response pattern has been shown across individuals and all age levels.[12]

Rats have been shown to habituate to repeated presentations of oral stimuli in the absence of gastric fill, demonstrating that the phenomenon does not rely on postingestive signals.[13] Research has also found that obese individuals habituate slower to repeated food stimuli than nonobese individuals.[14] Also, habituation has been found to be dependent on the hedonics of the food. If there is a liking or desire for the food, habituation for that food is slower to occur; conversely, a decrease in liking for the food is associated with a quicker habituation rate. These findings suggest that there is a specific sensory satiety component to the habituation of food processes.[15] It seems logical to conclude that unhealthy foods are probably more likeable and palatable and would thus produce a slower habituation rate than healthy foods. This slower rate to habituate to unhealthy food stimuli would cause an individual to eat more unhealthy than healthy foods. Electrophysiological evidence in rats supports this assumption. Research has found significant decrements in rats' neuronal responses in their brain reward centers with repeated food presentations that are modified by the presentation of a new food.[16] This finding implies that much of habituation to food stimuli is a product of the reinforcement value produced in the brain.

To remedy these maladaptive learned responses, one would want to retrain the body's rate of habituation to intense versus nonintense food stimuli as well as to "desirable and undesirable" foods. This retraining can be accomplished with deliberately measured portions on one's plate. In fact, one might want to consider using plates with preset dividers on it to pursue this retraining. If that person is involved in preparing his or her meal, prior to serving up the portions onto their plate, they should distinguish which food items they deem "most desirable, somewhat desirable, and least desirable." The food items that are deemed "least desirable" should then constitute the largest serving on that individual's plate. Preferably one would want to put those food portions in the largest divider section of the plate. Next, a smaller helping of the "somewhat desirable" item should be put in the smaller divider section of the plate. Finally, the food item deemed "most desirable" should constitute the smallest serving on one's plate.

Upon sitting down for the meal, one should have two goals in mind. First, consume large mouthfuls of the least-desirable food (to give a stronger intensity to the food and thus slowing down the habituation process to that food), while taking small mouthfuls at a time of the desirable food, lessening the intensity of the food and increasing its satiety rate. The second goal should be to consume all of the least-desirable food on one's plate. This exercise, if practiced consistently, will retrain the body's satiety rate with regard to desirable and least-desirable foods. Optimally, least-desirable foods will be consumed with such intensity and quantity that the body will learn to take longer to habituate to these foods and hold off sending satiety signals to the brain. Conversely, with desirable foods eaten in low intensity and smaller quantities, the body will learn to habituate quicker to these foods and send satiety signals earlier to the brain than in the past.

The concept of habituation can also be applied to the times that we are accustomed to having our meals. The old adage of having "three set square meals a day" may in part be a contributing factor to our bodies habituating to specific times throughout the day when food is expected. Consider children attending school who are accustomed to having their snack and lunch breaks at the same times each day. No doubt these students are developing a sense of regularity so that their digestive organs become habituated to begin the digestive process at certain times each day, whether food is present or not. Suppose no food is ingested at that set time; the digestive system will experience distress and hunger will occur. In this case, the cues of hunger are not physiologically based but preempted by learned behavior that most individuals are not aware that their bodies have learned. The cues of hunger will cause many individuals to mindlessly consume food, regardless if they are truly hungry or not.

Once a person becomes cognizant of this learned/habituated behavior, steps can be taken consistent with the habituation theory to extinguish the body's time-elicited hunger cues. To retrain one's body, put off eating that meal for an hour or two. The following day, the time of that particular meal should be varied from the previous day's time. This pattern should be followed for 3 to 5 days to extinguish the body's learned response of meal regularity. Due to being in a regimented environment (e.g., schools, work, military), however, this recommendation may not be possible for every person to implement. If this is the case, then it is recommended, if one is not experiencing "true hunger," to forego that meal until the next scheduled meal. This process, if executed every other or every third day, will give the digestive organs a rest, and simultaneously dishabituate the body from sending out hunger cues at specific times during the day. Optimally, if an individual could vary the times each day for each meal, the body would be less likely to send out cues of false hunger throughout the day and an individual would be less likely to waver from his or her eating plan.

Strategies to Counteract Classically Conditioned Eating Behavior

Classical conditioning is another form of learning that plays a role in our eating patterns. Our bodies can be easily taught that one stimulus can signal the occurrence of another stimulus soon to come. For example, if you visualize yourself eating a cupcake, according to the principles of classical conditioning, the body will initiate insulin secretion from the pancreas in preparation for the anticipated intake of sugar that would occur if you actually ate the cupcake. Hypothetically, then, if no sugar is eaten, the insulin secreted would lower the blood sugar level, causing an increased craving for a cupcake. In other words, instances of simply contemplating eating sweet foods can be a critical factor that sabotages an individual's strong resolve to limit these foods when following a particular eating plan.

Restaurants and other food establishments regularly utilize classical conditioning to increase sales of food. These establishments know that the odor of food is stimulating to the appetite so they use fans to arouse interest by people walking past the restaurant. The aroma of the food alerts the digestive system that food will arrive soon so the body physiologically begins to make preparations for the ingestion of food. When food is not ingested, the stomach sends distress signals to the brain until we act on those signals. Consider when you meet friends who are eating; you may not be hungry when you join them, but soon the odor and sight of the food will initiate a classically conditioned response. Similarly, seeing a magazine or television ad for food, even when an individual has just consumed a full meal, can trigger a classically conditioned response of hunger or salivation and cause an individual to eat foods that may not be included in their food plan.

INCORRECTLY ASSOCIATING FATIGUE WITH HUNGER

As you are undoubtedly becoming aware, we can become classically conditioned to associate almost any stimuli with another stimuli and respond accordingly. A common association that develops for many of us is the need for physiological rest and hunger. Many of us, upon feeling tired, incorrectly label this feeling as hunger. To our own detriment we eat instead when rest is really needed. Interestingly, digesting food requires energy thus making us more fatigued.[17] Simply being aware of this incorrect learned association between feelings of fatigue and hunger is half the battle. The principles of classical conditioning can also be used to extinguish this learned response. If an individual is feeling tired, they should take a 20-minute power nap to regain their energy. If they experience fatigue during the evening hours, they can move their bedtime up by an hour or so. If they are not in the position to rest, they can learn to take deep breaths to awaken the body by providing stimulating oxygen to their system. Another remedy would be to learn to drink a glass of water upon feeling tired. This new association between feelings of fatigue and a craving for water will rehydrate and energize the body. Whichever course of action they choose to use to respond to their fatigue, they need to make sure that the same response is consistently applied (e.g., deep breaths, a glass of water) in order to develop a new learned association between feeling fatigued and an appropriate and healthy proactive behavior. This new learned response will ensure that one is clearly identifying what their body needs (i.e., rest, not food) and will increase their success in adhering to their eating plan.

INCORRECTLY ASSOCIATING EATING WITH AN IMPROVED MENTAL STATE

Another incorrect association that can be learned is the association of a positive mental state with eating. Our mental outlook can be affected by our body's blood-sugar levels; when our body's blood-sugar level drops too low, depression tends to occur; when our blood-sugar level is at an optimum level, there is a feeling of well-being. Hence, a Pavlovian association with eating and well-being can incorrectly be developed. When we eat to provide stimulation, we disrupt the balanced mechanisms that would otherwise lead us to eat exactly the right foods in the right amounts. For every emotional high we experience, there follows a greater low. This association then develops into a vicious cycle of emotional ups and downs, undoubtedly disrupting our adherence to a healthy eating plan. Again, we can apply classical conditioning to undo this learned association. To extinguish this unwanted association, one can take a variety of paths. Upon feeling emotionally low, one should avoid reaching for foods that contain stimulants such as sugar or caffeine because these only provide a temporary surge of energy. Instead, choose to engage in a behavior that will improve the mood (e.g., talking about it with a close friend, looking at uplifting photographs, journaling).

If one consistently pairs these two concepts—low mood and uplifting activity—together, then the mind and body will come to realize that food does not provide a positive change to one's glum mental state. However, being engaged in an uplifting activity will not only improve one's mood but also will increase adherence to one's nutritional plan. Another alternative to erase the association between eating and happiness is to write down a list of positive events in one's life that one is thankful for. This method will cognitively shift one's mental framework to a more positive outlook. If this response is consistently executed when feeling emotionally down, then the body will eventually be retrained to look for a cognitive/mental solution as a mood enhancer instead of food.

Strategies to Counteract Operantly Conditioned Eating Behavior

Like classical conditioning, operant conditioning can be applied as well to any nutrition adherence plan. Operant conditioning, the process of behavior modification by which a subject comes to associate a desired behavior with a previously unrelated stimulus, can be easily executed and maintained throughout one's life if one follows the concept's tenets. For operational conditioning to work with regard to a healthy eating plan, one must have a beginning baseline behavior (e.g., eating 1 cup of vegetables per day), and an endpoint that they wish to achieve or maintain (e.g., eating 3 cups of vegetables per day). The key principle to operant conditioning with regard to nutrition adherence is making small changes in graduated steps over time. For instance if an individual is currently consuming 1 cup of vegetables per day and their goal is to consume 3 cups of vegetables per day, they may set an intermediate goal of consuming 2 cups of vegetables each day for 1 week. To accomplish this, they could choose to do one of the following: add 1 cup of salad to their dinner meal, eat 1 cup of baby carrots with their sandwich at lunch, or add 1 cup of steamed vegetables to their dinner meal. Any type of proactive change would be considered a form of effective behavior modification as long as it is a permanent change and not just a temporary change.

Next, to facilitate the change, operant conditioning utilizes rewards as reinforcement. Being rewarded for a specific behavior will increase the likelihood that one will perform that behavior again. However, the effectiveness of operant conditioning is contingent upon the manner in which the reinforcement is given. Reinforcement is most effective if implemented immediately after the changed behavior is exhibited. However, because food intake occurs over an entire day, one can implement the reward toward the end of the day and the reward will still have a strong effect. The most effective rewards are activities that one does often and loves to do already, whether it is watching TV, playing video games, going out with friends, or reading a magazine or book. Using rewards of favorite foods or snacks should be avoided. Consistent with the principles of operant conditioning, the reward should only be given each day that an individual meets their goal. However, if the individual fails to complete a day without following through with their changed behavior (goal), a reward must not be given. If a reward is given, the process of behavior modification will be completely negated.

Once the individual successfully completes an entire week with the modified behavior, they set an additional goal toward changing another part of their eating plan for the following week. For instance, now that they are successfully eating 2 cups of vegetables each day, they set a goal to eat 3 cups of vegetables each day for the following week. The steps they could take to achieve this might be to drink a glass of vegetable juice each morning for breakfast or add 1 cup of chopped vegetables to their sandwich at lunch each day. Again, the reward process would continue in the same manner as previously stated.

For formalized weight-management classes or sessions, operant conditioning could be used by having the participants earn points for every day they meet their eating behavior change goal and each time they complete an exercise session. Later, these points could be used to obtain a refund of their class fee or to pay for exercise classes. The behaviors being conditioned are the establishment of healthy eating habits and regular, consistent exercise, while the reinforcement is the refund of class fees or free exercise classes.

It is important to be aware that habits, good or bad, are formed by repetition. Eating habits are no exception. If Susan is in the habit of snacking while watching TV after work, Susan is reinforcing that habit until finally it becomes part of her regular routine. Other habits are formed in the same way. Some of these habits include eating while reading, eating the minute one comes in the house, eating when the children come in from school, eating when one comes in from a date, or eating while cooking dinner. As discussed earlier, certain moods and circumstances cause people to eat even if they are not hungry; for example, anger, boredom, fatigue, happiness, loneliness, the kids are finally in bed, nervousness, anxiety, or our spouse brings home candy or ice cream. All of these may trigger an eating response. Habits are hard to break. We must not only break these unhealthy habits, but we must set goals to form healthier habits in the same manner through repetition with an appropriate reinforcement.

Some Ideas for New Healthy Habits

1. Eat three meals a day. Have two or three preplanned snacks each day.
2. Prolong a meal by eating slowly, putting down the eating utensil between each bite, engaging in conversation, or taking sips of beverages between bites of food.
3. Choose a specific place in your home or at work to eat all of your meals and snacks.
4. Do not do anything (e.g., watch TV, read) except eat when you sit down for a meal or snack. Be mindful of the eating process (e.g., notice the smell of the food, the particular texture, flavors, temperature) in order to fully enjoy it.
5. Keep all food in the kitchen and do not store tempting foods where they are easily visible.
6. Do not buy junk food. Purchase plenty of fruits and vegetables for healthy snacks.
7. Serve food on smaller plates.
8. Substitute a snack each day for 20 minutes of exercise.

Note: As previously mentioned, the rewards given for a modified behavior need to be meaningful to the recipient.

Relevant reinforcement could be any of the following:

a walk	calling a friend	playing with the cat
writing or emailing a letter	reading a magazine or a book	cross-stitching
painting	gardening	surfing the Web
playing a favorite sport	walking the dog	listening to music
a long bath	woodworking	daydreaming
planning vacation	a cup of hot tea	looking at family pictures

You Diagnose It

ADHERENCE SCENARIO 1

Felicia's dietitian has advised her to keep a food log documenting times during the day, situations, and emotions that trigger her to eat foods that are not on her eating plan. After accumulating 1 week's worth of data, Felicia and her dietitian infer that she has difficulty adhering to her eating plan when:

(Continued)

a. She is sick, tired, or bored.

b. It is 10:00 AM.

c. She comes home from work.

d. She walks past a fast food restaurant.

   1. Use the concept of classical conditioning to explain how Felicia has been conditioned to have difficulty following her eating plan when simply walking past a fast food restaurant.

   2. Apply the concept of habituation to explain Felicia's difficulty in following her eating plan when it is 10:00 AM every day.

   3. Develop an operant conditioning adherence strategy to replace Felicia's need to eat when feeling bored, tired, or sick.

ADHERENCE SCENARIO 2

Lena is trying (though unsuccessfully) to eliminate soda pop from her daily eating plan. Each time that Lena goes a day without a soda, she rewards herself by treating herself the following day to a sweet treat. On those days when Lena indulges in just half a can of soda pop, she only treats herself to a small portion of a sweet treat the next day.

1. Based upon your knowledge of the operant conditioning theory, why is Lena's reinforcement plan ineffective?

2. How could Lena use the concept of classical conditioning to eliminate her craving for soda pop?

Review

✓ Researchers who take on the behaviorist perspective believe that the only way to know someone is to watch what he or she does—their behavior. The roots of the behaviorist perspective come from three philosophical ideas. One of the philosophical ideas comes from empiricism: the idea that all knowledge comes from experience. Behaviorism also comes from associationism: any two events, people, or objects that are repeatedly experienced together that become mentally considered as one and, thus, the person's reaction to one also becomes his or her reaction to the other as well. Lastly, behaviorism finds its roots in hedonism, the idea that people learn for two purposes: to seek pleasure and to avoid pain.

✓ Habituation is the simplest form of learning. After repeated exposure to the same stimuli, one habituates to it and over time stops responding to the stimuli.

✓ Classical conditioning/learning involves teaching an individual that one stimulus can signal the occurrence of another stimulus that is soon to follow.

✓ Operant conditioning is a process of behavior modification in which the likelihood of a specific behavior is increased or decreased through positive or negative reinforcement each the time behavior is exhibited.

✓ All three forms of learning (habituation, classical conditioning, and operant conditioning) can explain eating behavior and also be applied to learning proactive eating adherence behavior.

D.I.E.T. (Do I Eat This?)

TIPS TO CONSIDER WHEN REACHING FOR A PIECE OF FOOD

- Is this feeling I am experiencing true hunger or is it tiredness or perhaps another emotion?
- Am I eating while engaging in another distracting activity (e.g., watching TV, reading, emailing)?
- Will I receive a reinforcer at the end of the day if I engage in this eating behavior?
- Is this craving for food true hunger or a learned association with something in our environment?

REFERENCES

1. Ader, R. (1988). The placebo effect as a conditioned response. In R. Ader, H. Weiner, & A. Baum (Eds.), *Experimental Foundations of Behavioral Medicine: Conditioning Approaches* (pp. 47–66). Mahwah, NJ: Erlbaum.
2. Suchman, A.L., & Ader, R. (1992). Classic conditioning and placebo effects in crossover studies. *Clinical Pharmacology Therapy, 52,* 372–377.
3. Watson, J.B. (1930). *Behaviorism* (Rev. Ed.). New York: Norton.
4. Mickley, G.A., Kenmuir, C.L., Dengler-Crish, C.M., McMullen, C., McConnell, A., & Valentine, E. (2003). Repeated exposures to gustatory stimuli produce habituation or positive contrast effects in perinatal rats. *Developmental Psychobiology, 20,* 549–562.
5. Brickman, P., Coates, D., & Janoff-Bulman, R. (1978). Lottery winners and accident victims: Is happiness relative? *Journal of Personality and Social Psychology, 36,* 917–927.
6. Chance, P. (1988). *Learning and Behaviour.* Belmont, CA: Wadsworth.
7. Miller, W.R., & Seligman, M.E.P. (1975). Depression and learned helplessness in man. *Journal of Abnormal Psychology, 84,* 228–238.
8. Thorndike, E.L. (1911). *Animal Intelligence.* New York: Macmillan.

9. Skinner, B.F. (1938). *The Behavior of Organisms: An Experimental Analysis*. New York: Macmillan.

10. Swithers, S.E., & Hall, W.G. (1994). Does oral experience terminate ingestion? *Appetite, 23*, 113–138.

11. Ernst, M.M., & Epstein, L.H. (2002). Habituation of responding for food in humans. *Appetite, 38*, 224–234.

12. Colombo, J., Frick, J.E., & Gorman, S.A. (1997). Sensitization during visual habituation sequences: Procedural effects and individual differences. *Journal of Experimental Child Psychology, 67*, 223–235.

13. Swithers-Mulvey, S.E., Miller, G.L., & Hall, W.G. (1991). Habituation of oromotor responding to oral infusions in rat pups. *Appetite, 17*, 55–67.

14. Epstein, L.H., Paluch, R., Smith, J.D., & Sayette, M. (1997). Allocation of attentional resources during habituation to food cues. *Psychophysiology, 34*, 59–64.

15. Hetherington, M.M., & Rolls, B.J. (1996). Sensory-specific satiety: Theoretical frameworks and central characteristics. In E.D. Capaldi (Ed.), *Why We Eat What We Eat: The Psychology of Eating* (pp. 267–290). Washington, DC: American Psychological Association.

16. Rolls, E.T. (1984). The neurophysiology of feeding. *International Journal of Obesity, 8*, 139–150.

17. Segal K.R., Presta E., & Gutin B. (1984). Thermic effect of food during graded exercise in normal weight and obese men. *American Journal of Clinical Nutrition, 40*, 995–1000.

Chapter 3

Theories of Behavioral Change

LEARNING OBJECTIVES

By the end of this chapter, the reader will be able to:

1. Identify the three behavioral theories of change in nutrition adherence.
2. Identify the cognitive factors that lead to changes in eating behavior.
3. Apply the behavioral change strategies to a nutrition adherence program.

Mention Your Intentions

Server: Hello. Welcome to the Chart Club Restaurant; may I take your order?

Patron: Yes, I would like to order your Cobb salad with oil and vinegar dressing on the side.

Server: Excellent choice. Would you care for anything else?

Patron: Yes, when you bring me the salad, could you bring a to-go container with it so I can put half the salad in it and will not be tempted to eat the entire meal?

Server: Yes, I would be happy to.

(10 minutes later. . . .)

Server: Here is your salad and your "to-go" container. Would you like me to put half of your salad in it right now for you?

Patron: Yes, that would be great and I will eat this half on my plate. Thank you.

BEHAVIORAL CHANGE PROCESSES

This simple scenario illustrates the implementation of the theory of planned behavior by a patron at a restaurant. Once this patron publicly announced his or her intention to only eat half of the meal, the need to behaviorally follow through with that commitment instinctively becomes very strong, thus producing the intended behavior; in this case, eating a smaller portion. This, in essence, is the theory of planned behavior, which is one of the three behavioral change theories that will be introduced in this chapter. In the previous chapters, several situational/environmental factors (e.g., number of tablemates present while dining) were highlighted to show how they can affect eating behavior. In this chapter, you will become familiar with how cognitive processes (e.g., motivations, thoughts, intentions, and perceptions) can serve as the impetus to predicting behavioral nutrition changes and adherence. In particular, the following theories of behavioral change will be presented: planned behavior, social learning, and transtheoretical. You will learn how to adjust individuals' environmental, cognitive, and motivational factors with regard to these theories to bring about the desired change in eating behaviors.

THE THEORY OF PLANNED BEHAVIOR

The theory of planned behavior (TPB) states that when an individual's intentions are stable, intentions are more predictive of future behavior than past behavior. TPB was proposed by Icek Ajzen in 1985 and was developed from the theory of reasoned action that was proposed by Martin Fishbein together with Icek Ajzen in 1975.[1] According to the theory of reasoned action, if people perceive the suggested behavior as positive (attitude), and if they think their significant others want them to perform the behavior (subjective norm), this results in a stronger intention (motivation) and they are more likely to engage in this intended behavior. (See **Figure 3–1** for an illustration of the theory). A drawback to this theory is that there can be circumstantial limitations that interfere with the intentions leading to an actual behavior. For instance, a circumstantial limitation to having a healthy lunch may be the lack of healthy food left in one's refrigerator. Due to these limitations, Ajzen developed the TPB by adding a new dimension: perceived behavioral control. Control factors include both internal factors (such as skills, abilities, information, and emotions) and external factors (such as situational or environmental factors).

The concept of perceived behavioral control originates from the self-efficacy theory (SET) developed by Albert Bandura in 1977.[2] *Self-efficacy* is

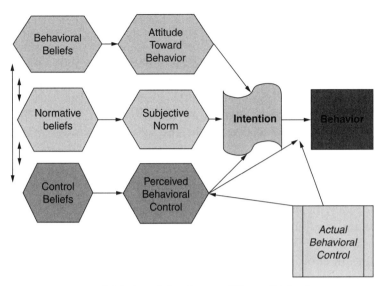

Figure 3-1 A Conceptual Display of the Theory of Planned Behavior.
Source: Adapted from Ajzen, I. (2002). Perceived behavioral control, self-efficacy, locus of control, and the theory of planned behavior. *Journal of Applied Social Psychology, 32,* 665–683.

defined as the conviction that one can successfully execute the behavior required to produce the desired outcome. Bandura states that self-efficacy is the most important component for any type of behavioral change because people's behavior is strongly influenced by their confidence in their ability to perform that behavior.[3] An individual's level of self-efficacy is usually measured with items that begins with the words, "I am sure I can, through self-report questionnaires. Ultimately what is being measured is an individual's confidence toward the probability, feasibility, or likelihood of executing a given behavior.

The concept of social influence plays a prominent role in the TPB. While most models are conceptualized within individual cognitive space, the TPB considers social influence, such as social norms and normative belief, based on collectivistic culture-related variables. Given that an individual's behavior (e.g., health-related decision making such as diet, weight management, and exercise) might very well be dependent on social networks and organizations (e.g., peer group, family, school, and workplace), social influence is a crucial element in the TPB.

Social influence is interpreted as the individual's elaborative thoughts on whether they are expected by their friends, family, and the society to perform the recommended behavior. Social influence is measured by evaluation of various social groups. For example, for weight loss:

1. Subjective norms from *peer groups* might include thoughts such as "Most of my friends are not overweight" or "I feel ashamed of my body in front of my friends who are not overweight."
2. Subjective norms from *family* include thoughts such as "All of my family members are overweight, and so it seems natural for me to be overweight too."
3. Subjective norms from *society or culture* include thoughts such as "Everyone else eats unhealthy meals too."

Essentially, the more favorable the attitude an individual has toward a behavior and a subjective norm and the greater the perceived behavioral control they have, the stronger the person's intention to perform the behavior in question should be. Ultimately, given a sufficient degree of actual control over the behavior, people are expected to carry out their intentions when the opportunity arises.[4]

The TPB has been applied to predicting human behavior in regard to several health-related fields such as condom use,[5,6] leisure,[7] exercise,[8] and of course diet.[9] The TPB model is thus a very powerful and predictive model for explaining human behavior. For instance, psychologists Mark Conner, Paul Norman, and Russell Bell published their research on TPB and healthy eating in the journal of *Health Psychology* in 2002.[10] One-hundred and forty-four patients attending health promotion clinics at their physicians' general practices were recruited into the study. The patients' intentions with regard to eating healthy, their current eating behavior, and their past eating behavior were measured over several months using a questionnaire format. At the conclusion of the study, the researchers found that people's intentions or consistent plans for engaging in healthy eating behavior were a predictive factor of their eating patterns, even 6 years after the study was conducted. In other words, stable intentions were more likely to be translated into subsequent action and healthy eating patterns, even when a person's past behavior (such as binge eating) was contradictory to the person's intentions.

Another study by Gardner and Hausenblas supports the utility and the predictive validity of the TPB for diet adherence.[11] In this 4-week long study, 69 women engaged in weekly exercise programs and a low-calorie diet. The researchers found that diet adherence as measured by the body mass index (BMI), circumference measurements, and weight was significantly predicted by the self-reported intentions construct of the TPB.

As previously stated, there are several components of the TPB that interact together to predict one's future eating behavior or the likelihood of an individual adhering to a specific food plan. The TPB can be expressed in the following mathematical function:

$$BI = (W1)\ AB\ [(b) + (e)] + (W2)\ SN\ [(n) + (m)] + (W3)\ PBC\ [(c) + (p)]$$

W = empirically derived Weights
BI = Behavioral Intention
AB = Attitude toward Behavior
(b) strength of each belief
(e) evaluation of the outcome or attribute
SN = Social Norm
(n) strength of each normative belief
(m) motivation to comply with the referent
PBC = Perceived Behavioral Control
(c) strength of each control belief
(p) perceived power of the control factor

Applying the Theory of Planned Behavior to Diet Adherence

Now that we are familiar with the TPB, let's apply it to predicting an individual's behavior with regard to weight loss. Consider Tricia's case:

Tricia is a 34-year-old woman who is married with three children all under the age of 7. Once a busy real estate executive managing two offices, Tricia is now a stay-at-home mother. Tricia is 5 foot, 7 inches and weighs 172 pounds with a BMI of 26.9. Before having her three children, Tricia weighed 123 pounds and had a BMI of 19.3 and was an avid runner. Tricia has expressed a desire to her physician to lower her BMI to 20.7 and to lose 40 pounds.

Will Tricia be successful attaining her goals? By implementing the TPB, we can predict the extent to which Tricia will achieve her goals. For now, we will focus on types of questions that measure each of the TPB constructs and what to do if Tricia's scores are low on a particular construct, thus decreasing the likelihood that she will stick to her reduced calorie food plan.

By using standard scaling procedures, we can assess the seven components of the TPB and more specifically Tricia's "attitude" toward weight loss, her subjective norms, her perceived behavioral control over losing the weight, and the strength of her weight loss intentions.

1. MEASURING DIET INTENTIONS

Here are some sample items that would be suitable to assess Tricia's weight loss intentions. (The respondent will circle the number that corresponds most closely to their current intentions).

- I intend to lose 6 pounds each month for the next 6 months.

  1   2   3   4   5   6   7   8   9   10

  extremely unlikely   extremely likely

- I plan to lose a total of 36 pounds over the next 180 days (6 months).

  1   2   3   4   5   6   7   8   9   10

  strongly disagree   strongly agree

2. MEASURING ATTITUDE TOWARD WEIGHT LOSS BEHAVIOR

Here are sample items to measure Tricia's attitude toward losing 36 pounds in the next 6 months.

- For me to lose 36 pounds in the forthcoming 6 months is:

  1   2   3   4   5   6   7   8   9   10

  harmful   beneficial

  1   2   3   4   5   6   7   8   9   10

  unpleasant   pleasant

  1   2   3   4   5   6   7   8   9   10

  worthless   valuable

3. MEASURING SUBJECTIVE NORMS TOWARD WEIGHT LOSS

Several different questions should be formulated to obtain a direct measure of Tricia's subjective norms. The following items illustrate the format these questions can take.

- Most people who are important to me think that

  1   2   3   4   5   6   7   8   9   10

  I should not   I should

     lose 36 pounds in the next 6 months.

- The people in my life whose opinions I value would

  1   2   3   4   5   6   7   8   9   10

  disapprove   approve

     of me losing 36 pounds in the next 6 months.

4. PERCEIVED BEHAVIORAL CONTROL OF LOSING WEIGHT

A direct measure of perceived behavioral control should capture Tricia's confidence that she is capable of performing the behavior of interest.

Some items have to do with the difficulty of performing the behavior or with the likelihood that the participant could do it.

- For me to lose 6 pounds in the forthcoming month would be

  1   2   3   4   5   6   7   8   9   10

  impossible   possible

- If I wanted to, I could lose at least 1.5 pounds per week in the forthcoming month.

  1   2   3   4   5   6   7   8   9   10

  definitely false   definitely true

5. WEIGHT LOSS BELIEF COMPOSITES

Beliefs play a central role in the TPB. They are assumed to provide the cognitive and affective foundations for attitudes, subjective norms, and perceptions of behavioral control.

By measuring beliefs, we can, theoretically, gain insight into the underlying cognitive foundation of why people hold certain attitudes, subjective norms, and perceptions of behavioral control. This information can prove very valuable for designing effective programs of behavioral intervention.

- Losing 1.5 pounds each week in the forthcoming month will lower my blood pressure.

  1   2   3   4   5   6   7   8   9   10

  extremely unlikely   extremely likely

6. MEASURING NORMATIVE BELIEFS ABOUT WEIGHT LOSS

The assessment of normative beliefs follows a logic similar to that involved in the measurement of behavioral beliefs. Assume that Tricia's family is one of the accessible referents.

- My family thinks that

  1   2   3   4   5   6   7   8   9   10

  I should not   I should

     lose 1.5 pounds each week in the forthcoming month.

- When it comes to losing weight, how much do you want to do what your family thinks you should do?

  1   2   3   4   5   6   7   8   9   10

  not at all   very much

Measures of normative belief strength and motivation to comply with respect to each accessible referent offer a "snapshot" of perceived normative pressures in Tricia's life.

7. MEASURING SALIENT CONTROL FACTORS

To generate a list of accessible factors that may facilitate or impede Tricia's behavior, the following questions can be asked.

- What factors or circumstances would enable you to lose 1.5 pounds each week in the forthcoming month?
- What factors or circumstances would make it difficult or impossible for you to lose 1.5 pounds each week in the forthcoming month?

Example: Assume that one of the accessible control factors has to do with work-related demands on time.

- I expect that my work will place high demands on my time in the forthcoming month.

  1   2   3   4   5   6   7   8   9   10
  strongly disagree   strongly agree
  Control belief power

- My work that places high demands on my time in the forthcoming month would make it

  1   2   3   4   5   6   7   8   9   10
  much more difficult   much easier

  to lose 1.5 pounds each week for the next 6 months.

EVALUATING TRICIA'S RESULTS

Once the likelihood of Tricia's diet adherence behavior is calculated (See www.people.umass.edu/aizen/tpb.html), go back and look at her individual scores on each of the seven constructs. If we find that Tricia is only 55 percent likely to exhibit the desired behavior, we can begin to play detective and determine which of the seven components of the TPB is negatively affecting her weight loss behavior. After looking over her self-report on the subjective norm measures, we might find that those individuals important to her do not support her or feel that she needs to lose weight. Here is a prominent stumbling block for her weight-loss behavior. At this point, a counselor, registered dietitian, or Tricia herself, would want to explore Tricia's perceptions in greater detail. Ultimately through self-analysis, family, and/or nutrition counseling, these subjective norms could be changed, thus increasing Tricia's likelihood of successfully achieving her weight-loss goal.

HOW MAKING A PUBLIC COMMITMENT EFFECTS OUR FUTURE BEHAVIOR

Suppose Tricia's responses to the previous questions reveal that she has about a 70 percent likelihood of sticking to her food plan and losing 1.5

pounds each week. How can we increase the likelihood of her exhibiting this behavior (in addition to adjusting any of the seven constructs of the TPB that might be low)? Psychological research has shown that people who have told others that they are on a diet are more likely to stick to their food plans for fear of appearing inconsistent to others. Why exactly does this occur? Dr. Robert Cialdini in his book *Influence: Science and Practice*, states that people have a natural desire to appear consistent with their words, attitudes, beliefs, and deeds.[12] Cialdini reports that this desire is due to three factors:

1. Good personal consistency is highly valued by society.
2. Consistent conduct provides a beneficial approach to daily life.
3. A consistent orientation makes it easier to make decisions with regard to our behavior.

In addition, Cialdini's research has shown that commitments are most effective when they are active, public, effortful, and viewed as internally motivated and not coerced. Once a stand is taken, there is a natural tendency to behave in ways that are stubbornly consistent with the stand. The drive to be and look consistent constitutes a highly potent tool of social influence, often causing people to act in ways that are clearly contrary to their own best interests.[13]

Examples of Public Commitment and Behavior Change

In his book, Cialdini gives one example of how public commitments make our behavior consistent. He noted that one restaurant was having problems with a large number of patrons who neither honored their reservations nor called to cancel them. Rather than take a hard-handed approach to solving the problem, the owner came up with a simple yet profoundly effective solution. The owner had the hostess change her usual request when taking a reservation over the telephone. Instead of saying "Please call if you have to change your plans," she rephrased the statement as a question. She began asking "Will you call if you change your plans?" The question caused the patron to commit to calling if they could not keep or needed to change their reservation. The no-show rate at the restaurant fell from 30 percent to 10 percent.

An example of public commitment and consistency involves a friend of the first author who volunteered for the March of Dimes. Several years ago, a caller from the March of Dimes' headquarters called and asked if Leah would be the volunteer for her neighborhood and send out donation cards to everyone on her street for the spring fundraiser. Leah told the caller that she would. On each of the cards that she distributed to her neighbors it said that she was a March of Dimes supporter and asked if they would contribute as well. There was also a place, on the letter to her neighbors, in which to sign her name. She did not realize it at the time that she had just committed herself publicly to be a lifetime supporter of the March of Dimes. Now whenever she sees a donation box at a grocery store for the March of Dimes, she instinctively drops her coins in. As you probably guessed, she says "yes" each year when they ask her to send donation cards out to her neighbors.

Let's go back to the scenario concerning Tricia. By using what we know about the TPB and concept of public commitment and consistency, it would be in Tricia's best interest to tell her coworkers, family members, friends, her trainer at the YMCA, the server at her favorite restaurant, her favorite cashier at the supermarket, her hairdresser, and her physician that she is making lifestyle changes in her eating habits. Tricia should not just tell these friends that she is on a reduced calorie food plan; she should share with them what she "intends" to accomplish. She should also give them a timeline and tell them specifically how she will do it. Too, she should let them know the reasons why she is going to do it. Believe it or not, people are fascinated with others' weight-control behavior—just look at all of the publicity tabloids give to celebrities about their weight gains and losses and the public buys it!

After telling everyone around her of her intentions, Tricia should keep them informed about her progress. No need to brag, but just let them know during those times of notable success about how well she is doing with her weight-management plans. Tricia should begin to see herself as a role model of healthy eating and living to others. She may even want to write—and sign—a gently worded contract for herself and post it near her computer or on the refrigerator. A sample contract might go something like this:[14]

> "I, Tricia Montgomery, promise to start today, February 21, 2010, to eat in a healthy manner. I promise not to indulge or gorge on foods that are unhealthy for me. I promise not to be caught up in the moment and reach for something sweet to restore my energy or take away my stress. I will be a paragon of healthy eating to myself, my family, and others. I also promise to treat myself gently if I ever stray from my commitment. These changes will help me to lose 1.5 pounds each week for the next 6 months."[15]

> Sincerely,
> *Tricia Montgomery*

The Need to Be Consistent and Its Effect on Our Behavior

Why is having a document in writing so important to honoring a commitment? The following is a wonderful example discussed in Cialdini's book to answer that question. During the Vietnam War, a different form of brain-washing was used by the enemy on American POWs. The technique did not involve any type of physical or mental torture, but involved commitment and consistency. The POWs were asked if they would like the opportunity to win a pack of cigarettes. Of course, many of them said yes. Their captors told them that they could write an essay and that the winner of the essay contest would win the pack of cigarettes. Each POW could write an essay about either the merits of communism or discredit communism in their essays. The captors would then award the best essay the prize. The captors also added that essays espousing the merits of communism sometimes had a higher likelihood of winning the contest. Many of the POWs wrote pro-communist essays—and what do you know, those POWs with the procommunist essays won the pack of cigarettes. The captors then sweetened the deal and told the winner that he could get an extra cigarette by simply signing his name to the essay. Most of the winners obliged to this offer. To carry the contest even further, the captors told the winner if he read his essay over the camp loudspeaker system, they would further sweeten the prize. Many POWs did just that and read their procommunist essay over the system, verbally espousing the merits of communism. When many of these essay contest winners were released from captivity, many elected by their own free will to stay in North Vietnam and embrace communism. How can that possibly be, you ask? Public commitment and consistency are the key factors at work here. Of their own free will, these men had written a viewpoint, signed their names to it, and then verbally espoused these views to everyone. They actually started to believe that they indeed favored the communist way of life; looking back at all of their freely chosen public actions reinforced this view. The effect of public commitment and consistency is a very effective phenomenon and is particularly beneficial when used to form healthy behaviors.

The Benefits of Making a Public Commitment

Another positive outcome of going public with your diet intentions is that the individuals who you interact with on a daily basis will be sensitive to your needs. The coworker whose desk is right next to yours will resist putting a jar of chocolate candy kisses on her desk to munch on. Your spouse will not be upset with you when you only eat half a portion of the meal that has prepared for dinner. Get the idea? Once everyone knows about your effort to change your eating behaviors, they will come forward and offer advice and encouragement or even help you to avoid "giving in" at the office party when the pizza arrives. When everyone knows about your plans, it is hard to back down and admit defeat because you feel that you will be letting yourself down—and everyone else as well.

TRANSTHEORETICAL MODEL OF CHANGE

The second psychological model of behavioral change that will be discussed in this chapter is the transtheoretical model of change.[16,17,18] This theoretical model integrates key constructs from other theories. This model of change posits that behavior change is a process, but not a linear process. It requires awareness over a period of time and many trials of the new behavior. The following are the steps of the stages of change in this transtheoretical model:

1. *Precontemplation:* The individual has no intention to perform the behavior (e.g., eliminate foods with high amounts of added sugars) and may not have even considered it.
2. *Contemplation:* The individual has formed an intention to perform the new behavior sometime in the future, but has not done so yet.
3. *Preparation:* The individual has a positive intention and makes some initial or occasional attempts to perform the behavior (e.g., sometimes using an artificial sweetener instead of real sugar).
4. *Action:* The behavior is performed consistently (e.g., limiting foods with high amounts of added sugars).
5. *Maintenance:* The individual persists in performing the behavior change consistently for a long enough time (6 months is suggested) that it becomes a regular part of one's routine and the probability of relapse to the former behavior is greatly reduced.

This model, like the TPB, involves emotions, cognitions, behaviors, and a reliance on self-report of the key constructs. The model has previously been applied to a wide variety of problem behaviors including weight control, exercise, low-fat diets, medical compliance, and smoking cessation.

Figure 3–2 illustrates how the temporal dimension is represented in the model. Two different concepts are employed. Before the target behavior change occurs, the temporal dimension is conceptualized in terms of behavioral intention. After the behavior change has occurred, the temporal dimension is conceptualized in terms of duration of behavior.

Regression occurs when individuals revert to an earlier stage of change. Relapse is one form of regression, involving regression from action or maintenance to a previous earlier stage. However, people can regress from any stage to an earlier stage. Some disheartening news is that relapse tends to be the rule

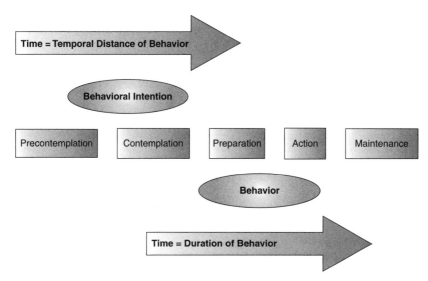

Figure 3–2 The Transtheoretical Model of Behavioral Change—The Temporal Dimension as the Basis for the Stages of Change.

Source: Adapted from Velicer, W. F, Prochaska, J. O., Fava, J. L., Norman, G. J., & Redding, C. A. (1998). Smoking cessation and stress management: Applications of the Transtheoretical Model of behavior change. *Homeostasis, 38,* 216-233.

when action is taken for most health-behavior problems. However, the upside is that not all people regress all the way back to the precontemplation stage. The majority of individuals regress to the contemplating or preparation stages.

The decisional balance scale involves weighing the *importance* of the pros and cons. A predictable pattern has been observed of how the pros and cons relate to the stages of change. **Figure 3–3** illustrates this pattern for eliminating sweets from one's diet. In the precontemplation stage, the pros of ingesting sweets far outweigh the cons of eliminating sweets. In the contemplation stage, these two scales are more equal. In the advanced stages, the cons outweigh the pros.

A different pattern has been observed for the acquisition of healthy behaviors. **Figure 3–4** illustrates this pattern for exercise. The patterns are similar across the first three stages. However, for the last two stages, the pros of exercising remain high. This probably reflects the fact that maintaining a program of regular exercise requires a continual series of decisions while eliminating eating sweets eventually becomes irrelevant. These two scales capture some of the cognitive changes that are required for progress in the early stages of change.

Self-efficacy can be represented by a monotonically increasing function across the five stages. Temptation is represented by a monotonically decreasing function across the five stages. Figure 3-4 illustrates the relation between stages and these two constructs.

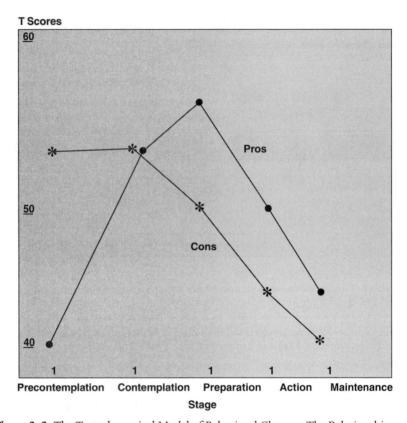

Figure 3–3 The Transtheoretical Model of Behavioral Change—The Relationship Between Stage and the Decisional Balance for an Unhealthy Behavior.

Source: Adapted from Velicer, W. F, Prochaska, J. O., Fava, J. L., Norman, G. J., & Redding, C. A. (1998). Smoking cessation and stress management: Applications of the Transtheoretical Model of behavior change. *Homeostasis, 38*, 216–233.

APPLYING THE TRANSTHEORETICAL MODEL TO DIET ADHERENCE

Now with a greater understanding of the stages that an individual passes through with regard to the transtheoretical theory, we can determine what stage of change an individual is at and then plan a course of action to propel them to the next progressive stage of change. For example, an individual who has been told by his physician to limit foods with large amounts of added sugar, but has not taken any course of action would be at the precontemplation stage. To propel this individual to the next stage, contemplation, one would want to increase the patient's sense of self-efficacy, while decreasing his environmental temptations. The patient's sense of self-efficacy could be raised by simply introducing him to artificial sugar substitutes, and his temptations lowered by removing foods from his home that contain

T Scores

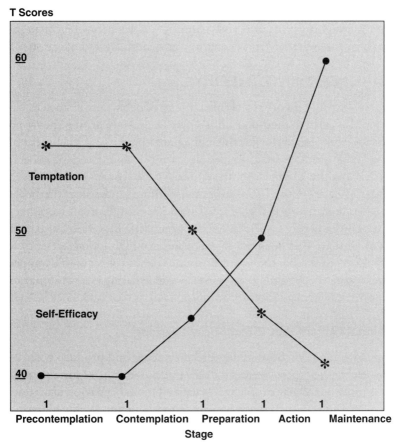

Figure 3–4 The Transtheoretical Model of Behavioral Change—The Relationship Between Stage and Both Self-efficacy and Temptation.

Source: Adapted from Velicer, W. F., Prochaska, J. O., Fava, J. L., Norman, G. J., & Redding, C. A. (1998). Smoking cessation and stress management: Applications of the Transtheoretical Model of behavior change. *Homeostasis, 38,* 216–233.

large amounts of added sugar. Also, at the precontemplation stage, the "cons" with regard to change in behavior will always far outweigh the "pros" of the behavior change. It would be advisable for the physician, registered dietitian, or nutrition counselor to sit down with the client and make up a list of the pros of limiting foods with large amounts of added sugar (e.g., calories utilized toward these foods can be used for more nutrient-dense foods, cravings for sweets may dissipate, can eat larger portions of other foods if concentrated sweets are reduced, etc.) and a list of the "cons" (e.g., can't eat what I want to eat when I want to eat it) of limiting foods with large amounts of added sugar. It is preferred to have more pros than cons in order to propel the client to the next stage of behavior change. As one can see the transtheoretical model of change revolves around changing an individual's cognitions (mentally weighing pros and cons) and his or her behavior through the increasing of self-efficacy and decreasing environmental temptations.

SOCIAL LEARNING THEORY

The social learning theory is the third theory of behavioral change to be discussed and applied to food-plan adherence. The social learning theory posits that people learn new behavior through reinforcement or punishment or via observational learning. Basically, people learn through observing others' behavior. If people observe positive, desired outcomes in the observed behavior, they are more likely to model, imitate, and adopt the behavior themselves. For instance, if you see a coworker eliminate salt from her diet and this consequently results in a reduction of her blood pressure, you are likely to emulate this behavior if you also have high blood pressure. This theory also suggests that the environment can have an effect on the way people behave. As the theory's name suggests, social learning is a combination of environmental (social) and psychological factors that influence behavior.

Additional Factors that Effect Social Learning

Social learning is not always guaranteed to occur and produce positive behavior. However, Albert Bandura (1977) outlined four requirements that make it more likely that people will learn and model behavior: attention, retention (remembering what one observed), reproduction (ability to reproduce the behavior), and motivation (good reason) to want to adopt the behavior.[19] Bandura points out that individuals are more likely to adopt a modeled behavior if it results in outcomes they value. Additionally, individuals are more likely to adopt a modeled behavior if the model is similar to the observer, has admired status, and the behavior has functional value. Bandura incorporates the previously discussed concept of self-efficacy into the theory in this manner: People are *more likely* to engage in certain behaviors when they believe they are *capable* of executing those behaviors *successfully*. This means that they will have high self-efficacy or self-confidence.

Bandura used preschoolers from the University's Stanford Bing Nursery School as his participants to illustrate social learning. In the study, each child viewed an adult either acting aggressively or nonaggressively toward a Bobo doll (an inflatable clown doll about the same size as a preschooler). Bandura found that after the adult had left the room, each child who had viewed the adult acting aggressively toward the blow-up doll would similarly engage in aggressive behavior toward the doll just as the adult had (e.g., hitting it with their fists or with a mallet). Those children who were in the condition in which the adult did not behave aggressively toward the doll did not hit the Bobo doll when the adult left the room. Bandura coined this type of learning as social learning or imitative or vicarious learning.[20] Bandura applied the findings of his studies to the effect that violence on television has on children's subsequent behavior, but we can very easily apply Bandura's social learning theory to nutrition behavior. For instance, if you see an individual exhibiting a certain type of behavior (e.g., eating in a healthy manner) and being rewarded for it (e.g., happy, upbeat mood, and a healthy looking physique), you will be more likely to emulate his or her behavior.

Researchers have also seen this occur in adults with diabetes who attend group nutrition education programs. In the program, participants learn how the amount of carbohydrate they consume affects their corresponding blood glucose levels. They are instructed to go home and eat a specific amount of carbohydrate and then test their blood glucose level. When they perform this activity, clients are able to see for themselves the direct correlation with diet (e.g., consuming less grams of carbohydrate at a meal) and their corresponding decrease in blood glucose levels. Once they return to the education program the following week, they share their findings with other group members. They inform the group that limiting their intake of carbohydrate resulted in the lowest blood glucose reading they have had in months. This positive response motivates other participants to change their diets in order to see if they will experience similar results by emulating the behavior of those who already have.

On the flip side, the social learning theory can work in the opposite direction. If you see someone exhibiting a certain behavior (e.g., indulging in unhealthy foods) and being punished for that behavior (e.g., unhealthy weight gain, not in good physical shape), you will not engage in that behavior. In the diabetes group just mentioned, some individuals will support this theory in that those who overindulge in carbohydrates will see an incremental increase in their blood glucose levels. They share this information with the group and group members will be less likely to engage in similar behaviors since it resulted in a negative outcome.

APPLYING THE SOCIAL LEARNING THEORY TO NUTRITIONAL ADHERENCE

When applying the social learning theory to a client's eating behavior, have your female client think through her life to someone she knew personally, who inspired her behavior in a positive way, then ask her, "Wouldn't it be wonderful to have a person like that to inspire you to adhere to your healthy eating plan?" Encourage her to find someone like that to serve as a mentor or role model. First, have her choose someone she knows personally and that she admires for his or her eating or exercise behavior. The client should let that person know that she admires them for that behavior. If she feels comfortable, talk to that person and solicit ideas as to what works for them. She should find out who inspired their behavior. If she feels very comfortable with them, she may ask to see their kitchen, refrigerator, and pantry for ideas on healthy food choices. Additionally, she should observe what they eat for a meal and their eating style. The client doesn't need to follow everything that the mentor does, but utilize the mentor to gather ideas that she likes and thinks will work for her and her lifestyle. If she is having trouble finding a mentor, she can look for a reputable authority figure instead, such as her physician or a registered dietitian.

It is amazing the lengths that individuals may go to in order to comply with the requests (e.g., healthy eating patterns, weight-loss requests) of authority figures. Advertisers commonly capitalize on this phenomenon. Dr. Robert Cialdini, in his book *Influence: Science and Practice,* illustrates this phenomenon with the marketing many years ago of Sanka decaffeinated coffee.[21] Robert Young, who played Dr. Marcus Welby on television, was given the job as the spokesman for this new product. Sanka sales then skyrocketed. Why? Television viewers associated Robert Young with his role of a doctor and considered him knowledgeable on the product that he was touting as better for our health than caffeinated coffee. Simply put, Cialdini states in his book *Influence*: "People rely on those with superior knowledge or perspective for guidance on how to respond and what decision to make."[22] You can probably think of more than a handful of television commercials that take place in a simulated doctor's office and feature an individual in a lab coat who is citing statistics. You may not be aware of it, but you are being unconsciously influenced to buy these products based upon the influence of the "authority principle" even if the authority figure is only an actor. To apply this phenomenon to nutritional adherence, seek out a credible authority figure (e.g., physician, registered dietitian, nurse) who can meet with you on a regular basis to provide support and advice.

Nutrition Experts

Registered dietitians, the nutrition experts, are trained to assist individuals in achieving their health and nutrition goals. They have a minimum of a baccalaureate degree in nutrition and related science courses. Upon college graduation, they are required to complete an internship and pass a national registration exam. Once they pass the exam, they are able to use the credential of registered dietician (R.D.) after their name. Registered dietitians can develop individualized weight-management plans that include goal setting, self-monitoring skills, and targeted nutrition education. Some dietitians complete additional coursework and training to specialize in the field of weight management. Registered dietitians can be located on the website of the American Dietetic Association at www.eatright.org, which is the professional association for registered dietitians.

| You Diagnose It |

ADHERENCE SCENARIO 1

Alex has just learned from the diagnostic tests that his allergist has performed that he is allergic to wheat. Alex's physician has told him to immediately eliminate all food products that contain any trace of wheat. Over the next 2 months, Alex tries to read the labels on the food products that he consumes to determine if they contain wheat. At restaurants—if he remembers—Alex will ask the server if wheat is used as an ingredient in any portion of the meal he intends to order. Despite these efforts, Alex still finds that he suffers from gastrointestinal discomfort from time to time due to the wheat that he unknowingly consumes in some meals.

1. What component(s) of the TPB could Alex utilize to increase his behavioral adherence to his wheat-free diet?
2. What stage of the transtheoretical model of behavior change is Alex at? What strategy could you implement to ensure that Alex moves onto the next stage of change?
3. According to the social learning theory, how would Alex learn to consistently eliminate wheat from his diet?

ADHERENCE SCENARIO 2

Marita has made a New Year's resolution to eliminate fast food from her daily eating pattern. Marita announced her resolution on January 1 to her husband and children at the breakfast table. Since then, Marita is having a difficult time adhering to her resolution. She finds that when she is short on time she will pick up lunch for herself and her family at a fast food restaurant.

1. Suggest how Marita could change some of her referent norms in life to allow her to increase her diet adherence behavior that would be consistent with the TPB.
2. Using the social learning theory, how could Marita learn vicariously to consistently eat healthy foods?
3. According to the transtheoretical model, which stage is Marita currently at? What strategy would a counselor implement so Marita does not regress back to the previous stage?

Review

✓ The theory of planned behavior (TPB) states that when an individual's intentions are stable, intentions are more predictive of future behavior than past behavior.

✓ The transtheoretical model of change posits that behavior change is a process, but not a linear process. It requires awareness over a period of time and many trials of the new behavior. The following are the steps of the stages of change in this model: precontemplation, contemplation, preparation, action, and maintenance.

✓ The social learning theory posits that people learn new behavior through reinforcement or punishment or via observational learning. Basically, people learn through observing others' behavior. If people observe positive, desired outcomes in the observed behavior, they are more likely to model, imitate, and adopt the behavior themselves.

D.I.E.T. (Do I Eat This?)

TIPS TO CONSIDER WHEN TEMPTED TO STRAY FROM MY FOOD PLAN

- What would my mentor do in this situation?
- Is eating this food consistent with my intentions and the eating behavior contract that I wrote and signed?
- By eating this food, will I be regressing back to a previous stage in the transtheoretical model?

REFERENCES

1. Fishbein, M., & Ajzen, I. (1975). *Belief, Attitude, Intention, and Behavior: An Introduction to Theory and Research.* Reading, MA: Addison-Wesley.
2. Bandura, A. (1977). *Social Learning Theory.* New York: General Learning Press.
3. Bandura, A., Adams, N.E., Hardy, A.B., & Howells, G.N. (1980). Tests of the generality of self-efficacy theory. *Cognitive Therapy and Research, 4,* 39–66.
4. Ajzen, I. (2002). Perceived behavioral control, self-efficacy, locus of control, and the theory of planned behavior. *Journal of Applied Social Psychology, 32,* 665–683.
5. Albarracin, D., Johnson, B.T., Fishbein, M., & Muellerleile, P.A. (2001). Theories of reasoned action and planned behavior as models of condom use: A meta-analysis. *Psychology Bulletin, 127,* 142–161.
6. Sheeran, P., & Taylor, S. (1999). Predicting intentions to use condoms: A meta-analysis and comparison of the theories of reasoned action and planned behavior. *Journal of Applied Social Psychology, 29,* 1624–1675.

7. Ajzen, I., & Driver, B.L. (1991). Prediction of leisure participation from behavioral, normative, and control beliefs: An application of the theory of planned behavior. *Leisure Sciences, 13*, 185–204.

8. Nguyen, M.N., Otis, J., & Potvin, L. (1996). Determinants of intention to adopt a low-fat diet in men 30 to 60 years old: Implications for heart health promotion. *American Journal of Health Promotion, 10*, 201–207.

9. Conner, M., Kirk, S.F.L., Cade, J.E., & Barrett, J.H. (2003). Environmental influences: Actors influencing a woman's decision to use dietary supplements *Journal of Nutrition, 133*(6), 1978.

10. Conner, M., Norman, P., & Bell, R. (2002). The theory of planned behavior and healthy eating. *Health Psychology, 21*, 194–201.

11. Gardner, R.E., & Hausenblas, H.A. (2004). Exercise and diet beliefs of overweight women participating in an exercise and diet program: An elicitation study using the theory of planned behavior. *Journal of Applied Biobehavioral Research, 9*(3), 188–200.

12. Cialdini, R.B. (2008). *Influence: Science and Practice* (5th ed.). Boston: Allyn & Bacon.

13. Ibid.

14. Blackman, M. (2008). Mind Your Diet: The Psychology Behind Sticking to Any Diet. Xlibris Corporation.

15. Ibid.

16. Prochaska, J.O., & DiClemente, C.C. (1983). Stages and processes of self-change of smoking: Toward an integrative model of change. *Journal of Consulting and Clinical Psychology, 51*, 390–395.

17. Prochaska, J.O., DiClemente, C.C., & Norcross, J.C. (1992). In search of how people change: Applications to addictive behavior. *American Psychologist, 47*, 1102–1114.

18. Prochaska, J.O., & Velicer, W.F. (1997). The transtheoretical model of health behavior change. *American Journal of Health Promotion, 12*, 38–48.

19. Bandura, A., Ross, D., & Ross, S.A. (1961). Transmission of aggressions through imitation of aggressive models. *Journal of Abnormal and Social Psychology, 63*(3), 575–582.

20. Ibid.

21. Cialdini, R.B. (2008). Influence: Science and Practice (5th ed.). Boston: Allyn & Bacon. References 55.

22. Ibid.

Section

II

COGNITIVE PROCESSES

Chapter 4

Attitudes and Eating Patterns

LEARNING OBJECTIVES

By the end of this chapter, the reader will be able to:

1. Understand how our attitudes drive human behavior.
2. Identify the three factors that comprise an attitude.
3. Identify processes that persuade us to change our attitudes.
4. Apply several relevant strategies to inoculate against counterproductive eating attitudes.

Some Asparagus Please. . . .

"No, thank you, I really don't like strawberry ice cream any more, but I will have some asparagus."

Can you believe you just made that statement? You are not alone in declaring your new aversion to ice cream and a love of asparagus, most of the other students who participated in the study at the University of California-Irvine, also have developed an aversion to ice cream.[1] How can this be? In one word, "priming." Priming refers to an increased sensitivity to certain stimuli due to prior experience—and the process takes place without our knowing it.

Some 200 student participants filled out questionnaires about foods and food memories. The next day, they were given the results of those surveys. Some results were true, while others were not. The experimenters fooled the participants with false computer generated information into believing that as kids strawberry ice cream had made them physically ill and that they, however, loved asparagus.

Those food memories were totally false and fabricated by the researcher for the study. However, many of the students internalized these memories as the truth and in follow-up food preference surveys, the students' food choices reflected their new attitude toward strawberry ice cream and asparagus. The mere belief that one had a negative food experience as a child is sufficient to influence food choices as an adult. Likewise, the (false) belief that one loved asparagus as a child is enough to positively influence that adult person to choose that food whenever possible.

As illustrated by Professor Loftus' study, individual perceptions and attitudes play a profound role in our daily eating patterns . . . sometimes without us even being consciously aware of it.

THE FIELD OF COGNITIVE PSYCHOLOGY

Another area of psychology that is very applicable to understanding our eating patterns is cognitive psychology. Cognitive psychology explicitly acknowledges the existence of internal mental states such as beliefs, desires, and motivations as fueling human behavior, unlike the behaviorist/learning perspective discussed in Chapters 2 and 3. Cognitive psychology is one of the more recent additions to psychological research. The field developed into a separate area within the discipline in the late 1950s and early 1960s following the "cognitive revolution" initiated by Noam Chomsky's 1959 critique of behaviorism, which was the dominant school of thought until that time.[2]

Traditionally, cognitive psychology includes topics such as human perception, attention, learning, memory, concept formation, reasoning, judgment and decision making, problem solving, and language processing. Some researchers have also included social and cultural factors, emotion, consciousness, animal cognition, and evolutionary approaches into cognitive psychology. For this chapter, the focus will be on three specific cognitive topics and how they affect eating behavior: attitude formation, persuasion, and resistance to attitude change.

ATTITUDE FORMATION AND CHANGE

An *attitude* is an individual's disposition to respond favorably or unfavorably to an object, person, institution, or event. Attitudes are judgments and are theorized to be made up of three components: affect, behavior, and cognitions (ABCs).[3] The affective component/response is an emotional response that expresses an individual's degree of preference for an entity. The behavioral intention is a verbal indication or typical behavioral tendency of an individual. The cognitive response is a cognitive evaluation of the entity that constitutes an individual's beliefs about the object.

Most attitudes are the result of either direct experience or observational learning from the environment. Attitudes can be changed in response to various stimuli, in particular persuasion. Carl Hovland, at Yale University in the 1950s and 1960s, helped to advance knowledge of persuasion.[4] Hovland theorized that we should view attitude change as a response to communication. He and his colleagues did experimental research into the factors that can affect the persuasiveness of a message. The following three factors are a product of Hovland's research findings.

1. **Target Characteristics**: There are qualities about the target person that will make him or her more or less likely to be influenced by the persuasive message. The influential characteristics of the person who receives and processes a message are intelligence and self-esteem; it has been found that more intelligent people are less easily persuaded by one-sided messages. Another variable that has been studied is self-esteem. There is evidence that the relationship between self-esteem and persuasibility is actually curvilinear, with people of moderate self-esteem more easily persuaded than both those of high and low self-esteem levels.[5] The mind frame and mood of the target also plays a role in this process.

2. **Source Characteristics**: Hovland also found that there are characteristics of the person delivering the message that affect its persuasibility. The influential characteristics of the source delivering the message are expertise, trustworthiness, and attractiveness. The credibility of a perceived message has been found to be a key component[6]; if one reads a report about health and believes it came from a professional medical journal, one may be more easily persuaded than if one thinks it is from a popular newspaper.

3. **Message Characteristics**: Last, the nature of the message was found to play a role in persuasion. Sometimes presenting both sides of a story helps to change attitudes.

A message can appeal to an individual's cognitive evaluation to help change an attitude. In the *central route* to persuasion, the individual is presented with the information, motivated to evaluate the information, and then arrives at an attitude-changing conclusion.[7] For example, an individual may be interested in losing weight and has tried a popular group-support program in the past without much success. They have a friend who has recently had success with a new group weight-management program and so they decide to attend an informational meeting for those interested in joining the program. At the meeting, they receive detailed information regarding how the program works, the cost, the various components, and so forth. As part of the presentation, they may also hear from a participant who has already been through the program and has experienced much success. Chances are, after they evaluate the information they have heard—particularly after hearing the success story—they may change their attitude about joining a group program and be the next participant to sign up.

In the *peripheral route* to attitude change, the individual is encouraged not to look at the content but at the source. An example of this would be a weight-management program that utilizes physicians to introduce the program to possible participants. If the physician, who is seen as a medical expert, endorses the program, participants are more likely to sign up. They may not even need to hear the specifics of the program. They believe that if the program is endorsed by a physician, then it has to be a good program. In addition to using physicians or other experts, this route to attitude change is also commonly seen in modern advertisements that feature celebrities or film stars. In this instance, they use their attractiveness or popularity to facilitate attitude changes. An example of this is when Oprah Winfrey followed a popular liquid diet utilizing a specific brand of milkshake-type drinks. She was very successful at losing weight by following this program and shared her success with viewers of her daytime talk show. Sales and demand for that particular weight program increased significantly after her show aired. People may have had a negative attitude toward liquid diets prior to viewing Oprah's show, however, they changed their attitude once they viewed her show and saw how successful she was in achieving her weight-loss goals.

EMOTION AND ATTITUDE CHANGE

Emotion is also a common component in persuasion and attitude change.[8] Emotion works tightly with the cognitive processes we use in various situations or when thinking about an issue. Emotional appeals are commonly found in advertising, health campaigns, and political messages. Current examples include smoking cessation health campaigns and political campaign advertising emphasizing the fear of terrorism.

Research suggests that persuasive fear appeals work best when people have high involvement and high efficacy. In other words, fear appeals are most effective when an individual cares about the issue or situation, and that individual possesses and perceives that they possess the agency to deal with that issue or situation.[9]

Important consequences of fear appeals and other emotion appeals include the possibility of reactance that may lead to either message rejections or source rejection and the absence of attitude change.[10] As the research suggests, there is an optimal emotion level in motivating attitude change. If there is not enough motivation, an attitude will not change; if the emotional appeal is overdone, the motivation can be paralyzed, thereby preventing attitude change.

Prominent factors that influence the impact of emotion appeals include self-efficacy, attitude accessibility, issue involvement, and message/source features. Self-efficacy is a perception of one's own human agency or our perception of our ability to deal with a situation.[11] For example, if a person is not self-efficacious about their ability to impact their own eating behavior, they are not likely to change their attitude or behavior about their diet.

Attitude accessibility refers to the activation of an attitude from memory or how readily available an attitude about an object or situation is.[12] Issue involvement is the relevance and salience of an issue or situation to an individual.[13] Past studies suggest accessible attitudes are more resistant to change.[14]

IMPLICITLY PRIMED ATTITUDES

There is also much research on implicit attitudes, which are attitudes unacknowledged or outside of one's awareness. These attitudes that lay in the subconscious portion of the mind are probably the most important determinants of our daily behavior and choices. We may not realize it, but the subconscious portion of our mind is being influenced or *primed* throughout each day as exemplified in the chapter's opening scenario. Once an individual's attitude is accessible to suggestion, it can be primed. Our minds are primed each day by many communicators and various forms of communication that can influence our attitudes and subsequent behavior without us even being aware of it. Priming is another technique that marketers use to influence food purchases and to increase consumption. Priming is used to evoke specific memories or associations that make a person more disposed to act in a particular way. Just as violent television programming can prime children to be more aggressive, sounds, smells, and also lighting prime people to be hungry or desire food. Mere exposure to a stimulus can influence attitude formation at below-conscious levels,[15] possibly because exposure frequency is experienced as affectively positive. [16] It should be noted that mere exposure and conditioning are concerned with attitude formation, not change.[17] This finding suggests that social marketing campaigns that associate positive role models with desirable behaviors (e.g., avoiding drugs or alcohol or eating healthy) might prove useful for those who hold neutral to positive initial attitudes toward the recommended actions.

SELF-PERSUASION–COGNITIVE DISSONANCE

So far we have discussed the mechanisms by which others can persuade our attitudes and subsequent behaviors. Now we are going to move into the realm of how our minds can become susceptible to self-persuasion and attitude change, otherwise termed as cognitive dissonance. Cognitive dissonance is an uncomfortable feeling caused by holding two contradictory ideas at the same time. The "ideas" or "cognitions" can include attitudes or beliefs and also the awareness of one's behavior. The concept of cognitive dissonance asserts that people have a motivational drive to reduce dissonance by changing their attitudes, beliefs, and behaviors, or by rationalizing their attitudes, beliefs, and behaviors.[18]

The state of dissonance typically occurs when a person perceives a logical inconsistency among his or her cognitions. For example, a belief in eating healthy could be interpreted as inconsistent with consuming a birthday cake. Becoming aware of the contradiction would lead to dissonance, which could be experienced as guilt, shame, anger, or any other negative emotional feeling. However, when people's ideas are consistent with each other, they are in a state of harmony or consonance.

A prominent cause of dissonance is when an idea conflicts with a fundamental part of one's self-concept of who they perceive themselves to be, such as "I am a good person" or "I made the right decision." The anxiety that comes with the possibility of having made a bad decision can lead to rationalization, the tendency to create additional reasons or justifications to support one's choices. A person with diabetes who just consumed a Danish might rationalize their guilt by believing that eating the Danish was necessary in order to provide them with the energy to get through their morning presentation at work. This belief may or may not be true, but it would reduce dissonance and make the person feel better. Because it is often easier to make excuses than it is to change behavior, dissonance theory suggests that humans are typically rationalizing while not always rational beings.

RESISTANCE TO ATTITUDE PERSUASION

After the Korean War with its incidences of brainwashing, psychologists tried to understand how to build up resistance to unwanted persuasion. McGuire and his colleagues proposed a technique called inoculation.[19] To inoculate an individual against persuasion, the person is exposed to weak attacks on a favored stance. The attacks must be weak so they do not truly change attitudes, but the individual is encouraged to fight them off and consequently learn to resist attacks. McGuire and his colleagues were able to show that, in these experimental situations, inoculation approaches were more powerful than simply telling a person that their opinion was right and that they should ignore attempts at persuasion.

Another technique that is similar to inoculation is forewarning, which is letting a person know ahead of time that their favored attitude will be challenged. This method allows a person to prepare to resist the message by rallying their defenses. If an individual is forewarned that a salesperson will call with a misleading offer, that individual is unlikely to find the salesperson persuasive.

THE APPLICATION OF ATTITUDE RESEARCH TO NUTRITION ADHERENCE

Our attitudes toward eating are made up of three components: affect, behavior, and cognitions. Each of these factors can affect or produce the other two factors. For instance, consider Jose's favorable attitude toward consuming carbonated soda pop. It could be viewing a positive emotion (affect) inducing advertisement for the soda pop that would instigate Jose's behavior of purchasing and imbibing the drink. After drinking the soda, Jose would make a cognitive assessment of that experience: "Wow, that tasted good." Or the attitude process could work in the opposite direction: after drinking (the behavior) a carbonated soda at a friend's house, Jose would produce the cognition, "I really liked the way that tasted," and then this cognition would produce positive affect. One can see that when exploring the origin of an eating attitude, one must investigate the directionality of the three ABC factors as illustrated in **Figure 4–1**.

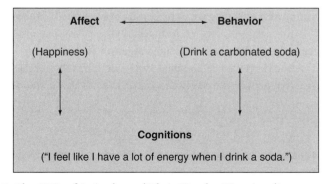

Figure 4–1 The ABCs of Attitudes and Their Circular Directionality.

When an individual is having difficulty adhering to a prescribed eating plan, it is prudent to uncover his or her attitudes toward the plan or toward the various subcomponents of the plan, as a starting place. Suppose Jenna is having trouble adhering to her goal of eating three servings of vegetables each day. A series of simple questions (**Figure 4–2**), with regard to her affect, behavior, and cognitions toward the plan would shed light on her adherence issues. A small (though not exhaustive) group of questions have been developed to illustrate the process of uncovering discrepant factors that make up one's attitude on a particular topic.

After examining the manner in which Jenna responded to each of the components comprising her attitude toward eating three servings a day of vegetables, we can see that her nonadherence lies within the cognitive component of her attitude, which ultimately affects her adherence behavior. Her maladaptive cognition that "It is difficult for me to prepare vegetables to eat each day" is the component of her attitude that is feeding her nonadherence behavior. Upon pinpointing this aspect, one would want to readjust or reform this maladaptive cognition through informed persuasion.

INDUCING CHANGE THROUGH THE PERSUASIVE SOURCE AND THE MESSAGE

As mentioned earlier in the chapter, our attitudes can be changed through direct or indirect experiences (e.g., books, advertisements, watching others). Additionally, the characteristics of the source delivering the message play a pivotal role in the effectiveness of the persuasive argument, because credible, attractive, and similar individuals to the target person are more likely to be persuasive. Now let's return back to scenario with Jenna and her difficulty in adhering to an eating plan that includes three servings of vegetables a day. By using a persuasive source and message, we can reformulate Jenna's cognitions so she will come to view vegetable preparation as easy. Careful consideration should be given when selecting who the persuasive source of information will be. Research would suggest that an individual who possesses similar characteristics to Jenna (or someone who Jenna can easily identify with) and who is attractive would be perceived as persuasive. Research has revealed that when it comes to attractive people, we apply the "what is beautiful is good" phenomenon to them or the "halo effect."[20] In other words, we assume that if a person is attractive, they must possess several other complementary traits (e.g., intelligence, kindness, credibility), and then we are more likely to be persuaded by the individual. Additionally, this individual needs to be perceived as a *credible* source of knowledge about nutrition or food preparation. For instance, because Jenna is a single mother of two small children who works full-time,

Affect Questions

1. I look forward to eating three servings of vegetables each day.

   1   2   3   4   5   6   7   8   ⑨   10
   Strongly Disagree   Strongly Agree

2. Eating vegetables is a very pleasant experience.

   1   2   3   4   5   6   7   ⑧   9   10
   Strongly Disagree   Strongly Agree

3. I like the taste of the vegetables that I choose to eat.

   1   2   3   4   5   6   7   8   ⑨   10
   Strongly Disagree   Strongly Agree

Behavior Question

4. I consistently eat three servings of vegetables each day.

   1   ②   3   4   5   6   7   8   9   10
   Strongly Disagree   Strongly Agree

Cognition Questions

5. I feel good about myself after eating three servings of vegetables a day.

   1   2   3   4   5   6   7   8   9   ⑩
   Strongly Disagree   Strongly Agree

6. I understand the importance of eating three servings of vegetables a day.

   1   2   3   4   5   6   7   8   9   ⑩
   Strongly Disagree   Strongly Agree

7. It is easy for me to prepare vegetables each day.

   ①   2   3   4   5   6   7   8   9   10
   Strongly Disagree   Strongly Agree

Figure 4–2 Questions to Determine One's Attitude Toward Change.

an ideal persuasive source would be another single, working mother with expertise in nutrition or cooking. If Jenna is presented with several persuasive arguments from another source who has no children or does not work, Jenna would be likely to discount their information on the grounds that the solution they offered would not work for her specific situation. For this situation, the source would perhaps show Jenna easy vegetable preparation techniques that have worked in her life (e.g., precut vegetables, tools that simplify the process).

Also, remember that presenting both sides to a persuasive message is very effective. Jenna's source may want to sympathize with her perception that preparing vegetables can be time consuming and difficult and present several reasons for that point of view. After she points out the potential difficulties, then she will make a case for the easy vegetable preparation techniques that she has developed. By presenting both sides of the argument, Jenna will feel that her initial cognition of "vegetable preparation as difficult" was indeed validated, and then be more receptive to other incoming information.

One would also need to consider which method to use when delivering the persuasive message to Jenna: the central route or the peripheral route of persuasion. Remember that when one uses the central route to persuasion, the information is presented and the target is given time to evaluate and process it. The peripheral route of persuasion, on the other hand (typically used in advertisements), emphasizes the source of the information, but not the content of the message. An infomercial for culinary tools that "slice and dice and make food preparation a breeze" would be an appropriate use of the peripheral route to persuade Jenna to reform her cognition that vegetable preparation can be quick and easy. However, a book written by an attractive, single, working mother titled *Food Preparation Shortcuts for the Hopelessly Busy Person* would represent using the central route to persuade Jenna.

INDUCING CHANGE THROUGH EMOTIONAL APPEALS

Suppose that Jenna's prior survey responses indicated that she did not understand the rationale for eating three servings of vegetables daily. In addition to the prior attitude change methods described, one could induce change through an emotional fear appeal. Remember that research indicates that persuasive fear appeals work best when an individual has high involvement in the issue at hand and perceives themselves as having a high level of self-efficacy. In other words, fear appeals are most effective when an individual cares about the issue or situation, and that individual perceives that they possess the abilities to deal with that issue or situation.[21] In Jenna's case, an emotional fear appeal might consist of visually depicting the physical consequences of not receiving the proper nutrients that three daily servings of vegetables would provide to her body. Graphic pictures of an individual who severely lacks these nutrients could be displayed to her as well as a list of the deleterious effects that this type of malnutrition will have on her brain and its daily processes. As the research reveals, this fear appeal will only be persuasive if Jenna cares about the issue at hand—her body—and has a sense of self-efficacy to bring about change to her situation.

Reactance, which occurs when an individual adopts an attitude that is contradictory to the one previously held because he or she perceives her behaviors are being limited or threatened, is the one issue to be aware of when using fear appeals to induce eating adherence. If the fear appeal campaign through the graphic photographs is unable to stir up an optimal level of emotional arousal in Jenna, then she will not be motivated to change her attitude. Likewise, if the appeal stimulates too much arousal within Jenna, she will become paralyzed with fear, thus not taking any action or believing that it is too late to take action. When presenting a fear-laced message, one must remember to strive to produce an optimal, manageable level of arousal within the recipient. Also, make sure that accessible information about courses of action that the individual can take to alleviate their current situation is provided within the message. Because many fear appeal messages are not delicately balanced in this manner, many message recipients are actually motivated to embrace their existing attitudes more strongly than ever.

INDUCING NEW ATTITUDES THROUGH THE PRIMING OF OUR SUBCONSCIOUS

Priming is another technique that marketers use to influence food choices and to increase consumption. Priming is used to evoke specific memories or associations that make a person more disposed to act in a particular way. This method of attitude formation takes place usually at the subconscious level without the recipient's awareness. Researchers employed the use of a liquor store to test their hypothesis that individuals' eating preferences can be influenced by a prime.[22] The researchers' hypothesis was supported as they found that patrons in the store were more likely to buy French wines when the store played French music and more likely to purchase German wines when German music was played.

Additional primes can be more subtle and priming can occur even through subliminal exposures. For instance, restaurateurs are now aware that playing slow music increases the time that people spend at their tables, while fast music increases turnover. Therefore, the type of music played can influence the amount of food patrons consume, because people consume larger quantities the more time they spend at a dinner table. Another study supported the concept of food priming with regard to participants' preferences for drinks.[23] In this particular study, people who were thirsty were asked to taste and rate an energy drink. Prior to consuming the beverage, they were exposed to subliminal images in which one group was shown a person smiling, the next group was shown a person with a neutral expression, and the third group was shown a person frowning. The images only lasted 16 milliseconds and could not be perceived by conscious awareness. However, the individuals who had viewed the smiling person consumed more of the energy drink and rated it more favorably than the other groups. Those who had viewed subliminal pictures of an individual frowning drank the lowest amount and rated it poorly.

THE NEGATIVE CONSEQUENCES OF SUBLIMINAL STIMULI: EATING ON AUTOPILOT

It is important to realize that the part of our brains that oversees conscious awareness is relatively small and can process only 40–60 bits per second, which is equivalent to a short sentence. Further, our entire cognitive processing capacity, which includes the visual system and the unconscious, is estimated to be 11 million bits per second.[24] Visualize the thinking capacity functions of the human brain as being separated into two components. One portion is cognitive and allows us to make carefully considered decisions, but it may be operating, on average, less than 5 percent of the time. The other portion, the unconscious, is responsible for impulsive, automatic decision making. This process happens rapidly and is based on limited signals or cues and information. This portion dominates cognitive decision making when there is too much information, or when a person is under stress, tired, or preoccupied. This unconscious portion of our brain is believed to function and direct our behaviors at least 95 percent of the time.[25]

As we know, people can only process a limited amount of information at one time and when they are overloaded, they will make decisions automatically, with no conscious thought involved. This fact is exemplified in a study in which participants were asked to choose between fruit salad and chocolate cake after memorizing either a two-digit or seven-digit number. Forty-five percent of the participants who memorized the two-digit number chose the chocolate cake, while in those participants who memorized the seven-digit number, 62 percent chose chocolate cake. Ultimately, what occurred was that the group memorizing the longer number had less available brainpower to carefully consider the items and resorted to following their impulses.[26]

Likewise, there is a limit to how many demands any person can respond to during a given time period. When our decision-making and reasoning resources are depleted, we usually choose the default option that requires no processing demands. Many times when it comes to food, the default options that we choose are items high in sugar and fat. As this impulse and decision are taking place at the subconscious level, we typically lack insight into this process and instead are misled into identifying other causes for our loss of self-control. Armed with this knowledge and insight, we can look back at those incidences when we did not adhere to our eating plan and see a pattern. At those times when we did not adhere to our eating plan, we were more than likely overloaded with information to process (e.g., stress, work overload) and thus we subconsciously resorted to going with our impulses and eating foods not in our best interests. During days or times in our life when information and stimuli are not overloading our information-processing mechanisms, we find that we are able to adhere to our eating plan.

With this information in mind, we need to be more cognizant of our eating environments and the amount of stimuli that they produce. A study by deCastro and colleagues exemplifies this point.[27] The study revealed that as the number of tablemates increases at your dining table so too does the number of calories that you consume. These results would suggest that our attention is focused on attending to our tablemates and thus depleting our remaining resources so we rely on our automatic impulses or priming factors for food choices and portions. Other activities such as watching television, driving a car, or reading while eating will likely produce similar consequences of stimuli overload and trigger primed or automatic impulse eating, thus causing nonadherence to an eating plan. Remember it takes more cognitive effort to refrain from eating and very little cognitive effort to engage in an instinctual automatic activity such as eating.[28] To prevent our minds from reverting to primes to guide our eating behavior, "mindful eating" is the key. Mindful eating can only take place when we ensure our eating environments are devoid of unwanted stimuli that would redirect our attention resources.

INDUCING AN EATING-RELATED ATTITUDE CHANGE THROUGH SELF-PERSUASION

The phenomenon of *cognitive dissonance* (a state of unpleasant tension one feels when one's attitude and behavior are incongruent) can work in one's favor to induce healthy eating behavior or just as easily produce poor eating choices. Upon feeling this state of unpleasant arousal, one is forced to alleviate it through self-persuasion, either by changing one's attitudes to match their behavior or changing their behavior to match their attitudes. When one chooses to change one's attitude (self-persuade oneself) to match the behavior is typically when our eating goals start to quickly unravel. Consider this example: Marvin's eating plan includes eating only uncooked fruits and vegetables with no preservatives added. At lunch, when Marvin inspects the lettuce for his salad, he notices that most of the lettuce is spoiled. Wanting to satisfy his growling stomach, Marvin looks in his freezer and finds a premade frozen vegetable meal. Marvin then pops the meal into the microwave for the recommended time. While waiting for the timer to ring, Marvin feels some mental tension about his upcoming behavior of consuming a preservative-laden cooked vegetarian meal. To release this tension, Marvin persuades himself that it is OK to consume frozen meals with preservatives once in a while because it would be wrong to let the existing meals in her freezer go to waste. Due to a state of cognitive dissonance, Marvin has just successfully persuaded himself and given himself permission to not follow his eating plan. It would have taken more cognitive effort for Marvin to refrain from taking the frozen meal out of the freezer and going to the grocery store to purchase a new head of lettuce. In other words, it is usually more difficult to change one's behavior to match one's attitude than it is to change one's attitude.

A study published in the *Journal of Consulting and Clinical Psychology*, however, illustrates how one can use cognitive dissonance to one's advantage when trying to adhere to an eating plan.[29] In the study, 481 female high school and college students who felt dissatisfaction with their bodies, but who did not have an eating disorder and were not obese were recruited for the study. The participants were then divided into four groups. In one of two experimental groups, termed the healthy-weight intervention group, the subjects learned about metabolism, nutrition, and exercise. They were encouraged to think carefully about what they ate, rather than going with an easy but unhealthy option (such as having a pizza delivered to the dorm instead of going to the cafeteria salad bar).

In the other experimental group, called the dissonance intervention group, counselors led participants through a script that was aimed to induce cognitive dissonance. In the study, the dissonance-group participants developed arguments against the thin standard and then role-played a conversation they might have with a younger girl to dissuade her from trying to attain the thin ideal. Next they took action against society's judgments of thinness by placing antithin-ideal posters in school restrooms. In addition to these two groups, there were two control groups in the experiment whose behaviors were not designed to control obesity or eating disorders. After meeting annually for follow-up sessions for 3 years, the participants' current behaviors and emotional states, as well as their risk of developing an eating disorder, were evaluated. After 3 years, both experimental groups showed a prominent difference from the control groups. In the healthy-weight group, there was a 61 percent reduction in the risk of developing an eating disorder and a 55 percent reduction in the risk of obesity; in the dissonance group, there was a 60 percent reduction in the risk of developing an eating disorder. This study illustrated how actively ensuring that one's behaviors and attitudes are congruent can facilitate adhering to one's eating plan. As we will see in the following section, the same mental and behavioral techniques that one uses to ward off a state of cognitive dissonance, can also be used to ward off a persuasive advertising message or person.

Resistance and Inoculation Against Persuasive Food Messages

Baseball's great "Sammy Sosa Is Powered by Pepsi!" What athletically minded person could resist reaching for a Pepsi when they know that Sammy drinks it? Or buying a box of Kellogg's Corn Flakes, because it is the official cereal of the National Hockey League? We are continually bombarded with dozens of persuasive food messages a day, whether is it via the television, radio, a billboard, in a magazine, or from a persuasive coworker offering his home-baked chocolate chip muffins. To fend off these persuasive advances, one should utilize the principles of inoculation and forewarning. Remember when inoculating an individual against persuasion, the person is exposed to weak attacks on a favored stance and that person is encouraged to fight them off and consequently learn to resist attacks. Inoculation takes active mental and physical power as well. One way to inoculate oneself again persuasive food offers is through role-playing various persuasive food scenarios. One scenario may be at a restaurant with the restaurant server wheeling a dessert cart up to the table to highlight the dessert menu. Another scenario might be turning down a close friend's offer to grab fast food for lunch. The more practice one has in developing arguments for adhering to his or her eating plan in their mental arsenal, the more effective they will be at resisting counterproductive food offers.

Forewarning, which is letting the target individual know ahead of time that their favored position will be challenged, helps to build up an individual's immunity against persuasive food offers. By forewarning that a person or advertisement will soon be challenging your position, you will have time to gear up and develop persuasive arguments as to why you are not yielding or changing your eating behavior. Verbally practicing arguments in favor of adhering to one's eating plan each morning while driving or doing household chores can greatly booster defenses against tempting, yet counterproductive food offers.

You Diagnose It

ADHERENCE SCENARIO 1

Juanita has been successfully adhering to her gluten-free eating plan for the past 2 months. However, she knows that this afternoon she will be faced with the annual office party potluck in which each of her coworkers has made a delicious dish, all of which are not on Juanita's eating plan. Juanita, of course, brought in a potluck dish that will allow her to adhere to her eating plan.

1. Use the concept of cognitive dissonance to explain why Juanita might feel obligated to indulge in the food not on her eating plan. How could Juanita use the concept of cognitive dissonance in her favor to adhere to her gluten-free eating plan?
2. Because Juanita is forewarned about the office party food situation, develop three successful arguments she could use on her coworkers' persuasive food offers at the party so she can adhere to her eating plan.

ADHERENCE SCENARIO 2

Juanita, from Scenario 1, has just watched a television infomercial hosted by a former swimsuit model, describing a cake decorating kit that "allows everyone to create masterful pieces of artwork" on their cakes. The kit is only $19.99 and includes four different types of cake mixes and an array of frosting colors. Juanita has always wanted to create beautiful cakes for others on their special occasions.

1. Describe two persuasive factors that the infomercial implements to persuade Juanita to buy the product and not adhere to her eating plan.
2. Describe which route of processing that the infomercial used to appeal to Juanita.

Review

✓ Cognitive psychology explicitly acknowledges the existence of internal mental states such as beliefs, desires, and motivations as fueling human behavior.

✓ An attitude is an individual's disposition to respond favorably or unfavorably to an object, person, institution, or event, or to any other discriminable aspect of the individual's world.

✓ Attitudes are judgments and are theorized to be made up of three components: affect, behavior, and cognitions (ABCs).

✓ The subconscious portion of our minds can be influenced or primed throughout each day. Once an individual's attitude is accessible to suggestion, it can be primed.

✓ Cognitive dissonance is an uncomfortable feeling caused by holding two contradictory ideas at the same time. To alleviate this feeling, an individual will either change their behavior to match their attitude or their attitude to match their behavior.

✓ To inoculate an individual against persuasion, that person is exposed to weak attacks on a favored stance.

✓ Another technique that is similar to inoculation is forewarning, which is letting a person know ahead of time that their favored attitude will be challenged. This method allows a person to prepare to resist the message by rallying their defenses.

✓ People can only process a limited amount of information at one time and when they are overloaded, they will make food choices impulsively because it takes less mental effort to rely on primes or impulses to direct their eating behavior.

D.I.E.T. (Do I Eat This?)

TIPS TO CONSIDER WHEN REACHING FOR A PIECE OF FOOD

• Am I in a state of cognitive dissonance? Am I changing my attitude about my eating plan to match my behavior?

• Am I eating while engaging in another distracting activity (e.g., watching TV, reading, emailing)? Am I eating mindlessly or mindfully?

• Am I purchasing this food that is not on my eating plan because I am relying on the peripheral route of persuasion?

REFERENCES

1. Bernstein, D.M., Laney, C., Morris, E.K., & Loftus, E.F. (2005). *Proceedings of the National Academy of Science, USA, 102,* 13724–13731.
2. Chomsky, N. (1959). A review of B.F. Skinner's verbal behavior. *Language, 35*(1), 26–58.
3. Fishbein, M.M., & Ajzen, I. (1975). *Belief, Attitude, Intention, and Behavior: An Introduction to Theory and Research.* Reading, MA: Addison-Wesley.
4. Hovland, C.I., & Weiss, W. (1951). The influence of source credibility on communication effectiveness. *Public Opinion Quarterly, 15,* 635–650.

5. Rhodes, N., & Wood, W. (1992). Self-esteem and intelligence affect influence-ability: The mediating role of message reception. *Psychological Bulletin, 111*(1), *156–171.*

6. Hovland, C.I., & Weiss, W. (1951). The influence of source credibility on communication effectiveness. *Public Opinion Quarterly, 15,* 635–650.

7. Petty, R.E., & Cacioppo, J.T. (1986). *Communication and Persuasion: Central and Peripheral Routes to Attitude Change.* New York: Springer-Verlag.

8. Breckler, S.J., & Wiggins, E.C. (1992). Emotional responses and the affective component of attitude. *Journal of Social Behavior & Personality, 8*(2), 281–296.

9. Witte, K. (1992). Putting the fear back into fear appeal: The extended parallel process model. *Communication Monographs, 59,* 329–349.

10. Brehm, S., & Brehm, J.W. (1981). *Psychological Reactance: A Theory of Freedom and Control.* New York: Academic Press.

11. Bandura, A. (1992). Exercise of personal agency through the self-efficacy mechanisms. In R. Schwarz (Ed.), *Self-Efficacy: Thought Control of Action.* Washington DC: Hemisphere.

12. Fazio, R.H. (1986). How do attitudes guide behavior? In R.M. Sorrentino & E.T. Higgins (Eds.), *Handbook of Motivation and Cognition,* Vol. 1. (pp. 204–243). New York: Guilford Press.

13. Zaichkowsky, J. (1985). Measuring the involvement construct. *Journal of Consumer Research, 12,* 341–352.

14. Fazio, R.H., & Williams, C. (1986). Attitude accessibility as a moderator of the attitude perception and attitude-behavior relations: An investigation of the 1984 presidential election. *Journal of Personality and Social Psychology, 51,* 505–514.

15. Bargh, J.A. (2007). *Social Psychology and the Unconscious: The Automaticity of Higher Mental Processes.* Philadelphia: Psychology Press.

16. Winkielman, P., & Cacioppo, J.T. (2001). Mind at ease puts a smile on the face: Psychophysiological evidence that processing facilitation elicits positive affect. *Journal of Personality and Social Psychology, 81,* 989–1000.

17. Cacioppo, J.T., Marshall-Goodell, B.S., Tassinary, L.G., & Petty, R.E. (1992). Rudimentary determinants of attitudes: Classical conditioning is more effective when prior knowledge about the attitude stimulus is low than high. *Journal of Experimental Social Psychology, 28,* 207–233.

18. Festinger, L. (1957). *A Theory of Cognitive Dissonance.* Evanston, IL: Row, Peterson.

19. McGuire, W.J., & Papageorgis, D. (1961). The relative efficacy of various types of prior belief-defense in producing immunity against persuasion. *Journal of Abnormal and Social Psychology, 62,* 327–337.

20. Nisbett, R.E., & Wilson, T.D. (1977). The halo effect: Evidence for unconscious alteration of judgment. *Journal of Personality and Social Psychology, 35*(4): 250–256.

21. Witte, K. (1992). Putting the fear back into fear appeals: The extended parallel process model. *Communication Monographs, 59,* 329–349.

22. North, A.C., Hargreaves, D.J., & McKendrick, J. (1997). In-store music affects product choice. *Nature, 390*(6656), 132.

23. Berridge, K.C., & Winkielman, P. (2003). What is an unconscious emotion? (The case for unconscious "liking"). *Cognition and Emotion, 17*(2), 181–211.

24. Dijksterhuis, A. (2004). Think different: The merits of unconscious thought in preference development and decision making. *Journal of Personality & Social Psychology, 87*(5), 586–598.

25. Dijksterhuis, A. (2004). Think different: The merits of unconscious thought in preference development and decision making. *Journal of Personality & Social Psychology, 87*(5), 586–598.

26. Ferraro, R., Shiv, B. & Bettman, J.R. (2005). Let us eat and drink, for tomorrow we shall die: Effects of mortality salience and self-esteem on self-regulation in consumer choice, *Journal of Consumer Research*, 32(1), 65–75.

27. deCastro, J., & Brewer, E.M. (1992). The amount eaten in meals by humans is a power function of the number of people present. *Physiology Behavior, 51*(1), 121–125.

28. Bargh, J.A., & Chartrand, T.L. (1999). The unbearable automaticity of being. *American Psychologist, 54*, 462–479.

29. Stice, E., Shaw, H., Burton, E., & Wade, E. (2006). Dissonance and healthy weight eating disorder prevention programs: A randomized efficacy trial. *Journal of Consulting and Clinical Psychology, 74*, 263–275.

Chapter 5

Perception, Visualization, and Eating Patterns

LEARNING OBJECTIVES

By the end of this chapter, the reader will be able to:

1. Understand how our sense of perception and expectations can affect the foods we choose, their tastes, and the portion sizes.

2. Identify the perceptual biases that can cause us to incorrectly perceive ourselves and our eating environments.

3. Understand how the process of visualization works to create reality in our minds and our eating behavior.

4. Apply relevant perceptual and visualization strategies to adhere to an eating plan.

"So How About Some Green Ketchup for Your Fries?"

No, you did not read that wrong—green ketchup. Food companies have long known that consumers can be influenced by the use of food dyes to make food look more appealing, but researchers at the H.J. Heinz Company deliberately developed a colored ketchup that goes against our expectations of what the sweet condiment should look like. Heinz developed the EZ Squirt ketchup line that included ketchups in green, pink, orange, teal, and even blue. Heinz believed that these unexpected ketchup colors would get kids to change their perception of ketchup and get excited about the condiment, thus taking it out of the refrigerator more often. This marketing campaign worked for several years before it was terminated.

In addition to the unexpected colors, the nozzle on the container was designed to produce a thinner stream of ketchup that didn't splatter. The new bottle also used a softer plastic that was easier for small hands to squeeze. The goal of the people at Heinz was to make ketchup use fun for kids so they would create art projects with the ketchup and slather more of it on their foods.

Heinz certainly did their marketing homework, because prior to the design change, they spent a great deal of time with children in their homes and schools to gather their ideas on ketchup. What they observed was that the ketchup bottles were too big for little hands; mothers would typically take the bottle away from their children because they were afraid of the children making a mess.

With that information in hand, Heinz went to work on a better design. The ketchup researchers also asked the children for their thoughts on how to make ketchup more fun. One resounding idea was "turn it into a fun color"—which they did. Taste tests with children revealed that the funky-colored ketchup did not change their taste perception of the product. The end result was that households were more likely to buy two bottles of ketchup at the store, a "boring" bottle for adults and the funky-colored EZ Squirt bottle for their children. Pure marketing genius!

THE PROCESS OF PERCEIVING OUR ENVIRONMENT

In Chapter 4, we glimpsed the expansive field of cognitive psychology; in particular, how our attitudes shape our behavior. Another vital component to the field of cognitive psychology is the process of perception, which is closely related to attitudes. Perception is the process by which we interpret and organize sensations to produce a meaningful experience of the world.[1] In other words, when a person is confronted with a situation or stimuli, the person interprets the stimuli into something meaningful to him or her based on prior experiences. Sometimes, however, what an individual interprets or perceives may be substantially different from reality. The perception process typically consists of three stages: selection, organization, and interpretation.

Selection

A person's awareness and acceptance of the stimuli play a key part in the perception process. Receptiveness to the stimuli can be highly selective and may be dependent on a person's existing beliefs, attitude, motivation, and personality characteristics.[2] Individuals are known to attend to the stimuli that satisfies their immediate needs (perceptual vigilance) and may ignore stimuli that might create psychological anxiety (perceptual defense). Broadbent explained the concept of perceptual vigilance with what he called the filter model.[3] Broadbent believed that due to limited capacity, a person must selectively process information. However, when confronted with information from two different stimuli channels (i.e., methods of delivery such as visual and auditory), the individual's perceptual system processes the information that he or she deems as relevant. The perceptual defense system creates an internal barrier that limits the external stimuli passing through the perception process when it is not consistent with the person's current beliefs, attitudes, or motivational drives; this process is known as selective perception. Selective perception occurs when an individual limits the processing of external stimuli by selectively attending to what he or she sees based on beliefs, experience, or attitudes.[4]

Broadbent's filter theory has been added to over the years. A selection for action view posits that filtering is not just a consequence of processing limitations, but is driven by goal-directed actions.[5,6,7] The assumption is that any action requires the selection of certain aspects of the environment that are action relevant and, at the same time, filtering other aspects that are action irrelevant. Ultimately, when one is working toward a goal, one will bypass information that does not support one's goal.

> *The mind can only see what it is prepared to see.*
> —Edward de Bono

Organization

The second stage of the perception process—organization—consists of arranging the selected data in a meaningful way. We might organize data by its appearance, its interaction style, by our expectations, or even by using a stereotype. One's perception of the stimuli is dependent on what one believes he or she will see—or what they have been primed with.

Interpretation

The last stage of the perception process is the interpretation stage, in which we attach meaning to make sense of the data. The type of meaning that we attach can be dependent on various factors, such as our past experiences, beliefs, expectations, motivations; our knowledge; our degree of involvement; our self-concept; cultural factors; and of course our gender roles. For instance, what do you see in **Figure 5–1**? If you are in a good mood you might see

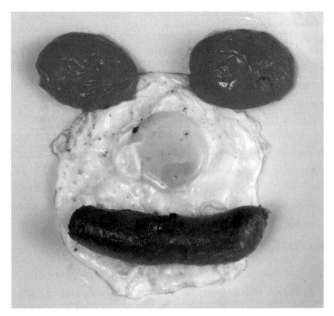

Figure 5-1 The Effect of Expectations on Perception.
Source: © Paul Cowan/Dreamstime.com

a happy face. However, if you are hungry, you might interpret it as breakfast with an egg and sausage. Keep in mind that all stages of the perception process can be affected as well by physiological processes such as fatigue, hunger, age, health, senses, and biological cycles. After completing the interpretation stage, we will either be prompted to take action or refrain from action.

ERRORS IN THE PERCEPTION PROCESS

Errors in the perception process can occur in any one of the three stages of the process. There are several biases that can potentially affect the accuracy of our judgments, however, we will discuss three biases in particular that are most relevant to our perceptions of our eating environments: the primacy effect, the contrast effect, and the mere exposure effect.

Primacy Effect

You are probably familiar with the saying "first impressions are lasting impressions." This adage applies in the perceptual process as well and is referred to as the primacy effect. Simply put, the object or stimuli that you are presented with first in a series of objects or stimuli is the one that you are most likely to remember the best. The phenomenon is due to the fact that the short-term memory—at the beginning of whatever sequence of events is being presented—is significantly less crowded. Because there are far fewer items being processed in the brain at this time, there is more time for rehearsal or pondering of the stimuli which can cause them to be transferred to the long-term memory for permanent storage. This phenomenon typically occurs during the "selection" stage of the perception process and can cause us to unintentionally take notice and remember trivial information, and subsequently discard more important information that is soon to follow.

Contrast Effect

Another type of bias in the perception process that can occur is a contrast effect. Contrast effects generally occur in the interpretation stage of the perception process and are tied to an individual's interpretation of stimuli based on comparisons with other stimuli that rank higher or lower on the same characteristics. For example, Wedell and colleagues found that, if compared to a highly attractive person, a target person of average attractiveness is perceived to be less attractive than he or she would have been if rated on his or her own.[8] Simply put, the contrast effect relates to how an object or individual is perceived in relation to others around it. An accurate interpretation of the stimuli is more likely to occur when no other comparison stimuli are present to influence the process.

The Mere Exposure Effect

The exposure effect (also known as the mere exposure effect or familiarity principle) is a phenomenon in which people tend to develop a preference for things merely because they are familiar with them. In studies of interpersonal attraction, the more frequently a person is seen by someone, the more pleasing and likeable that person appears to be—assuming that their first meeting was not negative. This phenomenon can be applied to various venues of stimuli such as music, consumer products, and food. For instance, the more times that you hear a new song on the radio, the more you are apt to like it. In other words, familiarity breeds liking. The mere exposure effect takes place both in the selection stage and the interpretation stage of the perception process. The repetition of the stimuli causes us to take greater notice of the stimuli and choose to process it; the repeated exposure causes us to interpret the stimuli in a positive light.

VISUALIZATION

One can recreate all of the stages of the perception process by implementing mental imagery, also known as visualization. *Visualization* is defined as an experience that resembles a perceptual experience, but which occurs in the absence of the appropriate stimuli for the relevant experience. Therefore, whenever we imagine ourselves performing a behavior in the absence of physical practice, we are said to be applying imagery. Although this discussion of mental imagery will focus mostly on the visual mode, there also exist the auditory and kinesthetic forms of visualization.

Visualization's Applications in the Field of Sports Psychology

Much of applied psychological research on visual imagery has been directed toward the area of sports. Many sports such as golf, tennis, and skating require not only physical skills, but a strong mental game as well. You have probably heard the adage that "sports are 90 percent mental and only 10 percent physical." This saying rings true in sports where hundredths of a second or tenths of an inch distinguish the champions from the commonplace athletes. To get that extra edge, numerous athletes incorporate mental imagery into their training regimens to take their game to the next level. Athletes typically use mental practice for improving their confidence, controlling their arousal levels and for performance preparation. These techniques can be easily applied to the field of nutrition and eating behavior as well.

There is no right method to implementing mental imagery. It can be done in any context such as on or off the field, for short or long duration, while lying down or sitting up. For example, a tennis player may use a few moments to visualize herself hitting the perfect serve in the place where she wants the ball to land. A quarterback can go through a play in his mind just before calling the play.

Isaac's sports-oriented study supports the effectiveness of mental imagery and future performance.[9] Isaac tested 78 participants and then categorized them as novice or experienced trampolinists. Next, she divided the two groups into an experimental and control group. She also divided the subjects up into either high or low imagers based on initial skill level. Both groups were trained in three skills over 6 weeks. The experimenter was blind to which group was the imaging group. The experimental group physically practiced the skill for 2.5 minutes, which was then followed by 5 minutes of mental practice. Finally, an additional 2.5 minutes of physical practice followed the mental practice. At the same time, the control group physically worked on the skill for 2.5 minutes, which was then followed by

5 minutes of a session trying a mental task of an abstract nature, such as math problems and puzzles Then, 2.5 additional minutes were spent physically working on the skill. The results of the study revealed that there exists a significant difference in the improvement of the high and low imagers. In both the novice and experimental groups where the initial skill ability was similar, the high-imagery groups showed significantly more improvement than the low-imagery group. In addition, there was a significant difference between the experimental and control groups. As one would surmise, the experimental group had significantly more improvement than the control group. This study indicates that despite the level of skill visual imagery can be very effective.

Additional support for the effectiveness of mental imagery can be found in a study by Roure and associates.[10] In this study using the sport of volleyball, Roure and colleagues found six specific autonomic nervous system (ANS) responses that correlated with mental rehearsal, thus improving sports performance. The subjects were placed in an experimental/imagery group and a control group. The task for each group was their ability to pass an opponent's serve to a given teammate. The experimenters measured the variations of the ANS during the motor skill and during the mental rehearsing sessions. The ANS indicators tested included skin potential and resistance, skin temperature and heat clearance, instantaneous heart rate, and respiratory frequency. The results of the test revealed a strong correlation between the response in the actual physical tasks (both pre and posttest volleyball) and during the mental imagery sessions. Ultimately, the mental imagery group possessed significantly stronger skills than those in the control group. In addition, no clear difference was present between the pre- and posttests in the control group. This study revealed that mental imagery induces a specific pattern of autonomic response, which included decreased amplitude, shorter duration, and negative skin potentials when compared to the control group. As a consequence of the ANS, the imagery group was associated with better performance. From the results of this study, Roure suggested that metal imagery may help in the development of schema which can be reproduced, without thinking, in actual practice.

Porter and Foster theorizes that the reason visual imagery works is that when you imagine yourself perform a task perfectly, you are physiologically creating neural patterns in your brain, just as if you had physically performed the intended action.[11] These patterns are like small tracks engraved in the brain cells that can ultimately enable an athlete to perform physical feats by simply mentally practicing the action. Thus, mental imagery is intended to train our minds and create the neural patterns in our brain to teach our muscles to do exactly what we want them to do.

Another domain that mental imagery has been found to enhance is that of intrinsic motivation. A study by Martin and Hall tested who would spend more time practicing a golf putting task and who would have higher levels of self-efficacy.[12] Thirty-nine beginner golfers were grouped into an imagery or control group. Both groups were taught how to hit golf balls for three sessions. The imagery group practiced in an imagery training session designed for that specific golf skill. As a result, the imagery group spent significantly more time practicing the golf putting task than the control group. Additionally, the subjects in the imagery group had more realistic self-expectations, set higher goals to achieve, and adhered more to their training programs outside the experimental setting than did the control group of golfers. As one can see from these studies, mental imagery is very effective in producing intended behaviors. Shortly, in the application portion of this chapter, we will apply the concept of mental imagery to the domain of eating behavior.

THE PROCESS OF PERCEPTION AND ITS EFFECT ON EATING-PLAN ADHERENCE

Eye-Catching Food

The process of perception, is at the heart of much of our eating behavior. In this section we will break down each of the stages of the process of perception and relate it to how it can affect our decision to eat a piece of food or forgo eating that particular food item. Let's look at the selection stage of the perceptual process in which the stimuli needs to catch the eye of the target individual in order to be considered for processing.

It is no secret that the way food looks plays a large part in our willingness to eat it. This assertion is backed up by the fact that outstanding chefs spend a large portion of their time perfecting the presentation of their plates. Additionally, food companies spend billions of dollars to put their food in the ideal light thanks to marketing and packaging strategies. In other words, top chefs and food companies are pandering to the selection stage of the perception process through these strategies; they are hoping through their clever methods, you will notice their product. For example, marketing researchers have shown that when the amount of shelf space in grocery stores for an item is doubled, sales of that item increase by 40 percent.[13,14] This effect occurs whether the item is generally popular or unpopular. Sales also increase when special displays and end-aisle displays are used and when items are placed at eye level.[15] Grocery chains aware of this principle maximize their revenue by arranging large, prominent displays of high-profit items, thus increasing the item's perceptual salience and the likelihood that you will process it further.

To further illustrate the effect that salience has on eating behavior, consider Wansink and associates' study with office employees in the workplace.[16] Wansink and his colleagues placed either transparent or opaque jars of chocolate candy Hershey's Kisses on coworkers' desks. Wansink showed that office workers ate 3.1 times more chocolate Kisses (total of 75 kcal) when the candy was placed on their desks in transparent jars than when the candy was placed in opaque jars. The adage "out of sight, out of mind" can sum up these results nicely. When a food item is not salient, it has a decreased likelihood of being recognizing by the perceiver and processed further. Further processing to the organization and interpretation stages might result in consuming the item.

However, if the food item does not register to our senses, then further processing is highly unlikely. One can see that because food is made salient to us numerous times a day through multiple venues (e.g., TV, magazine advertisements, grocery stores, billboards, radio), it is very difficulty to resist further processing of the food stimuli. If one were to apply the selection principle to help regulate our eating behavior, then one would want to limit the salience of food items not on one's eating plan and enhance the salience of those foods on one's eating plan. This could be accomplished by putting all foods not on one's eating plan out of sight in the cupboards or refrigerator, while putting those foods on one's eating plan on the counters in plain sight. A large bowl on the dining room or kitchen table filled with an assortment of fresh fruit is a good example of how to enhance the salience of healthier snack foods. Also, limiting one's exposure to food advertisements (fast forwarding through commercials on television or purposely avoiding the junk food aisles in grocery stores) would help to eliminate any salient food stimuli catching one's eye.

Easy-Access Foods

The next two stages of the perceptual process are the organization and interpretation stages of the stimuli. As mentioned earlier, the organization and interpretation of the stimuli is dependent on a person's existing beliefs, motivations, or emotional state (Assael, 1995).[17] For instance, we might process, organize, and interpret a peanut butter sandwich differently if we are hungry at the time of viewing it versus if we are feeling full. Viewing a peanut butter sandwich on an empty stomach would cause it to be highly salient to the perceiver, thus actively attended to, and then organized and interpreted as a stimulus that would satisfy an immediate need.

However, suppose the perceiver was not hungry at the time of being exposed to the sandwich. In this case, the sandwich may not even reach the first stage of selection of stimuli to be attended to in the perception process due to the perceiver's state of being satiated.

Research also suggests we are more likely to eat foods that we organize and interpret as easily accessible (e.g., ones that require the least effort to eat such as precooked and prepackaged foods that can be eaten without utensils). Incidentally, the foods that have shown the greatest increase in sales in the past quarter century are consistent with this idea: soft drinks, salty snacks, french fries, and pizza.[18] This principle, however, can also be used to encourage the intake of healthier food items such as fruits and vegetables. In today's grocery stores, consumers can find prewashed, precut, fruits, vegetables, and salad greens. Utilizing these easily accessible food items can make a significant difference in helping one to successfully adhere to their prescribed food plan.

Another study by Painter and associates exemplifies the principle that "as the effort to eat food decreases, the amount of food consumed increases."[19] This group's study revealed that office workers who had chocolate Kisses within reach on their desks ate an average of 5.6 more candies (total of 136 kcal) per day than did workers for whom candy was placed on a shelf 2 meters away. An even more compelling study illustrating this point was conducted by Wansink & Kim. Researchers found that the urge to eat food that is close by is so strong that human beings eat more even if the food tastes bad. A study at a movie theater where people were given 14-day-old popcorn in boxes twice the normal size illustrates this point. Patrons complained about the taste, but surprisingly still ate 34 percent more popcorn than did people given stale popcorn in boxes that were the normal size.[20] From this study, we can see that when food is easily accessible, our brains are more likely to perceive it and process it, which ultimately facilitates the possibility that we will eat that particular item of food.

Portion Size

The amount of food that we consume is also dependent on the organization and interpretation stages of the perception process. Consider these findings. A report by the Centers for Disease Control states that women eat 335 more calories a day than they did 30 years ago.[21] Part of this large intake increase can be attributed to something called portion distortion. You may not realize it, but your organization and interpretation of perceptions as to what constitutes a normal portion of food have changed over the past 20 years and have become greatly distorted. A study out of Rutgers published in the

September 2006 issue of the *Journal of the American Dietetic Association* reports that over the past 20 years, consumers perceive large portion sizes as appropriate amounts to eat at a single eating occasion.[22] This study replicated a study that was conducted over 20 years ago in which participants were asked to serve themselves the amount they considered to be a typical portion of each meal item from a buffet table. Schwartz and coauthor, Carol Byrd-Bredbenner, had 177 young adults participate in this study. Each participant was asked to attend one meal and select typical portions from a buffet of a total of eight meal items at breakfast or six at lunch and dinner. The portion sizes that the participants chose were significantly larger than the portion sizes chose in the study conducted 20 years prior, signifying that our perceptions of appropriate portion sizes have been dramatically exaggerated.

Interestingly, most foods with drastically different portion sizes over the two decades were all served and consumed from a cup or bowl. For example, typical portions of orange juice were more than 40 percent larger in the present day study than they were 20 years ago. This larger amount of orange juice provides 50 additional calories and could equal a 5-pound weight gain over a period of 1 year if consumed daily. The participants in the present study served themselves almost 20 percent more cornflakes and poured almost 30 percent more milk on their cereal than participants 20 years ago.

Interestingly, people who are served larger portions simply eat more food, regardless of their body weight and regardless of the food item, meal setting, or timing of other meals.[23,24,25] For example, patrons at a restaurant who were served a pasta dish that was 50 percent larger than the typical portion ate 43 percent more than people served the normal portion of the dish, increasing their caloric intake at the meal by 159 kcal.[26] Additionally, men given 175 gram bags of potato chips tripled the amount of chips they ate in comparison with men given 25 gram bags of potato chips, consuming an extra 311 kcal.[27] In another study conducted by Wansink and associates, a set number of soup bowls were connected to tubes hidden beneath a table which continuously fed tomato soup into the bowls. Participants in the study were assigned either to a regular bowl or the hidden automatic refillable bowl and told to eat the soup until they felt full. Those whose bowls were being automatically refilled consumed 75 percent more soup than those eating soup from regular bowls. One participant with the refillable bowl, when asked if he was full (after he had consumed close to a gallon of soup), looked down at his bowl that was still half full and said, "Why would you think I was full? I still have half a bowl to go."[28]

From these studies it is evident that we are becoming passive eaters who allow others to determine portion sizes for us. We need to counteract our incorrect perceptions as to what constitutes a normal portion size. We can learn to change the way that we "organize" food stimuli in the perception process. One way to do this is to learn what a normal portion size is for various foods on one's eating plan. A serving of a food item may be defined in several different ways depending on the food plan followed. For example, one serving can be the amount of food that food manufacturers list on the nutrition facts panel of food packages. The government also has defined standard serving sizes of food items based on consumer nutrition surveys. Too, one serving can be the amount of one food item from the various food groups on the U.S. Department of Agriculture (USDA) food guide pyramid.[29] For instance, the food guide pyramid defines 1 ounce of grain as a serving. One ounce of grain would be equivalent to 1/2 cup of brown rice or a 1 ounce slice of bread. Fruits and vegetables are measured in cups so if 2 cups of fruits are recommended, two household measuring cups of fruits should be consumed. Meat and protein servings are measured by ounce equivalents. One ounce of meat, fish, chicken, or other protein food is a piece about the size of a matchbox. Someone following a reduced calorie food plan of 1,500 calories would require about 5 ounces of meat/protein per day. Therefore, a dinner of a boneless, skinless, chicken breast weighing 3 ounces would be equal to three 1-ounce equivalents. The person would have 2 ounces or two "matchbox" 1-ounce equivalents left for the remainder of the day.

On the other hand, a portion of food is that amount of food that the person, another individual, or in some instances, the restaurant, may determine is appropriate. A portion of spaghetti at one restaurant may be 3 cups but at another restaurant a portion of spaghetti may be 6 cups. In a study conducted by Young and Nestle, nutrition students were asked to bring to class a "medium"-sized bagel, potato, muffin, apple, or cookie. The foods were then measured and weighed. Almost all of them exceeded the standard portion sizes as determined by the USDA.[30] In addition, our culture typically "super sizes" portions that further confuses the issue of what constitutes an appropriate quantity of food to eat.

To better estimate appropriate portions of foods, we can use common household objects to visualize a portion of food. For example, a 3-ounce portion of meat is equal to the size of a deck of playing cards. If, on a reduced calorie food plan, you are aiming to eat about 5 ounces of protein per day (as recommended by the USDA food guide pyramid), then you would aim to eat one piece about the size of a deck of cards and another piece slightly smaller than a deck of cards. If a 1/2 cup of carrots are equal to a scoop of carrots about the size of a tennis ball, you then know that you should be eating about four "tennis ball" amounts of vegetables per day in order to meet the USDA guidelines of 2 cups of vegetables per day. Likewise, if a 1-cup portion of fruit is about equivalent to a closed fist, you then know that you should eat at least two "fists" of fruit per day in order to meet the USDA guidelines. These visual food portion templates help to organize incoming food stimuli and facilitate our "interpretation" of correct portion sizes. They also can assist individuals in staying within a prescribed number of calories while still consuming a well-balanced and adequate food plan.

Food Expectations

Most of us would agree that taste is the most important sense when it comes to enjoying food, but how important is our perception or sight of the food? Try this perceptual experiment: Imagine that a bowl of yellow-colored gelatin is placed in front of you. How would you assume it will taste? You might think it will taste sour, because of your past experience with other yellow foods that are sour such as lemons and grapefruits. Or maybe you might think it will taste sweet, because of yellow sweet foods that you have tasted like bananas or pineapple. We have developed these kinds of taste associations through the years based on our prior experiences. Food advertisers use these associations to help sell their products and can change their customers' perception of how products will taste by manipulating their coloring. They go to extreme lengths to find the perfect mouth-watering color for their items because they know when it comes to taste, color does matter.

A study in the1970s found that the color of food had a significant effect on people's appetites.[31] Participants were placed in a room with special colored lighting and then given a plate of steak and French fries to consume, which looked normally colored. Then, the researcher changed the lighting to reveal to the participants that the steak was blue-colored and the fries were green. After realizing the food's true hue, some participants became ill. The reaction of these participants can be chalked up to our instinctual aversion to certain colors of food, with blue and purple as the prominent aversive colors. Keep in mind that blue and purple colors don't occur very often in natural foods, and in fact are sometimes associated with spoiled and moldy food. With this expectation affecting our interpretation stage of the perception process, we will interpret that foods of this color won't taste good or will be bad for us and choose not to eat them.

On the other hand, specific colors can enhance our enjoyment of food because we have associated the taste of a food with a color, even if it differs from that food's natural color. A prominent example of this association is butter, which in its natural state is almost white, but for commercial purposes is dyed yellow to look more appealing. The green Heinz ketchup in the chapter's opening scenario is an example of how color can positively affect the perception process in food consumption.

However, an unsuccessful example of this type of marketing was the development of Crystal Pepsi in 1992. The colorless, caffeine-free cola failed to become popular because many people could not make the connection between the cola's colorlessness and its taste. It was difficult for consumers to imagine a cola being clear, and some even claimed it tasted like lemon-lime soda. Through these relevant examples we can see how a food's coloring can greatly affect the interpretation stage of the perception process and ultimately the consumer's decision to eat the food or not.

PROMOTING EATING ADHERENCE BY AVOIDING PERCEPTUAL ERRORS

The primacy effect is a perceptual bias that can lead us to eat foods not on our eating plans. Consider perusing a restaurant's menu. Typically, we will read a menu's contents from left to right. Generally, high-caloric appetizers are the first food that you encounter on the menu and due to the primacy effect are the foods that you would be most likely to remember and order. Healthier foods and side orders are typically listed near the middle or end of the menu. Strategically, searching first for those healthy items on your eating plan will ensure that those items are the first ones that you process on the menu and thus will be more likely to order. Likewise, when shopping at a grocery store, the first items that you are likely to encounter—thanks to marketing manipulators—are high-calorie baked goods or prepackaged snacks. Upon encountering these items first, you are likely to think about them throughout your entire trip in the store and thus will have a higher likelihood of purchasing them. How do you avoid laying your eyes on these items first upon entering your local store? Know your grocery store! Strategize the healthiest entrance route to your grocery store. Enter the store through the door that leads to the produce section, so the first foods that your eyes see are fruits and vegetables. Shop the perimeter of the store where the produce, poultry, dairy, and eggs are located. Limit purchases from the aisles in between because this is where most all of the packaged and processed food items are located.

The contrast effect is another perceptual error that can lead to overeating. Remember back to Chapter 2's discussion of the concept of habituation, in which we become accustomed to or habituate to the taste of a food the more we consume it in one sitting. The food soon will lose the zest that we experienced in the first few bites that we took of it. In order to keep that taste sensation going, we generally try one of two things: We ingest large quantities of that food item in each mouthful or choose an alternate, but very similar, food item to replace that food sensation. The latter option successfully reproduces that original taste explosion due to the contrast effect.

Suppose you were eating a brownie for dessert and experienced an explosion of rich chocolate in your mouth upon the first bite. You notice upon finishing the brownie that the original taste explosion in your mouth is no longer occurring. You instinctively reach for another sweet treat, a chocolate chip cookie, in hopes of replicating that chocolate taste explosion. Due to the contrast effect, you perceive that this cookie is even sweeter than the last few bites of your brownie and you continue to ride the wave of this new taste explosion, eating more than you should. This pattern of overeating occurs due to an unfair comparison to a food that we have become habituated to and a new food that in contrast seems like it is zestier than the original food item. Though, if we had eaten one bite of each of these foods on two different days, we would have rated the chocolate brownie as much sweeter than the chocolate chip cookie. The key is to not get to the point in which you habituate to a specific food during a sitting. You can do this by serving yourself a small portion of that food, so when you finish the food, you have not habituated to it and then start the search of finding a substitute food to reenact that taste explosion, that the contrast effect promotes.

The last perceptual bias to be cognizant of when eating is the mere exposure or familiarity effect. Marketing experts rely on repeated exposure of their food items through advertisements to increase their appeal and sales. Assuming our first exposure to a new food product is neutral, all subsequent encounters with it will increase our desire for it. Limiting repeated exposure of food items not on one's eating plan is crucial to eliminate the effectiveness of the exposure effect. This can seem like a colossal task as we are bombarded with advertisements through numerous venues daily, but there are some proactive strategies that we can take to reduce its vice within our home environments. Prerecord all of your television shows during the week so that you can skip through the advertisements and not be subjected to repeated exposure of food stimuli. Consider your commute to work. Does your route pass by streets consisting of numerous fast food restaurants? If it does, change your route and take a different one that passes by a residential neighborhood instead. This way you are not being repeatedly exposed to foods not on your eating plan. Think about the magazines that you subscribe to. Do they have repeated advertisements for unhealthy foods? Try subscribing to a different type of magazine so you are not subjected to this repeated stimulus. Making small changes in your home environment will make a significant difference in your ability to successfully adhere to an eating plan.

VISUALIZATION AS A MEANS TO PROMOTING NUTRITION ADHERENCE

We have become familiar with the process of food perception and perceptual errors that can occur. We turn now to recreating that process within our minds in the absence of any real stimuli. This process, referred to as visualization or mental simulation, can provide a glimpse to the future by enabling people to envision possibilities and develop plans for bringing those possibilities to fruition. In moving oneself from a current situation toward an envisioned future one, the anticipation and management of behaviors are fundamental tasks as well as envisioning successful completion of a goal that involves a focus on self-regulatory processes. For example, if one has the goal of sticking to a reduced-calorie eating plan, then the visualization process can facilitate adherence to this plan. Ideally, one should start each day with the visualization process. Take time before rising out of bed to visualize each meal starting with the preparation process to its consumption. During the visualization process, one should only invoke images of adhering to his or her eating plan.

You can also visualize incidents in which others might offer you food that is not on your eating plan and you successfully push it aside. By consistently visualizing successful adherence to your eating plan, the mind will perceive it to be reality and in the presence of real food stimuli, the adherence behavior will have a higher likelihood of becoming routine and replicated in this environment. Visualization of resisting tempting food offers will also facilitate adherence to an eating plan. Just as we plan out each day before we go to school or work, so too should we plan out and visualize our eating behavior.

You Diagnose It

ADHERENCE SCENARIO 1

Gabe has been successfully adhering to a low-calorie eating plan for the past 4 weeks. However, Gabe has a business dinner meeting at an upscale restaurant tomorrow night. Gabe has not eaten out since he began his eating plan and is worried that he will succumb to ordering and eating foods that are not on his plan.

1. How could Gabe implement the process of visualization to ensure that he successfully adheres to his eating plan at the business dinner?
2. How might the server at this restaurant use the primacy effect to persuade Gabe to order and eat foods not on his eating plan?

ADHERENCE SCENARIO 2

Kathy and her husband enjoy traveling the world via cruise ships. The only problem is that they end up returning home with a weight gain of 5 to 8 pounds. Kathy attributes the weight gain to the beautifully crafted buffets on the ship that have several varieties of every type of food that you could imagine.

1. Describe how each of the three stages of the perception process are contributing to Kathy eating foods from the buffet that are not on her eating plan.
2. Explain how the contrast effect could potentially contribute to Kathy eating foods from the buffet that are not on her eating plan.

Review

- ✓ Perception is the process by which we interpret and organize sensations to produce a meaningful experience of the world.
- ✓ The perception process typically consists of three stages: selection, organization, and interpretation.
- ✓ Errors in the perception process can occur in any one of the three stages of the process. There are three biases in particular that are most relevant to our perceptions of our eating environments: the primacy effect, the contrast effect, and the mere exposure effect.
- ✓ The primacy effect occurs when the object or stimuli that you are presented with first in a series of objects or stimuli is the one that you are most likely to remember the best.
- ✓ The contrast effect relates to how an object or individual is perceived in relation to others around it.
- ✓ The exposure effect (also known as the mere exposure effect) is a phenomenon in which people tend to develop a preference for things merely because they are familiar with them.
- ✓ Visualization is defined as an experience that resembles a perceptual experience, but which occurs in the absence of the appropriate stimuli for the relevant experience.

D.I.E.T. (Do I Eat This?)

TIPS TO CONSIDER WHEN REACHING FOR A PIECE OF FOOD

- Am I eating this food simply because it is easily accessible?
- Has repeated exposure to this food that is not on my eating plan caused me to develop a preference for it?

- Am I consuming this food simply because it was the first food that I encountered on the menu or at the grocery store?
- Is eating this food consistent with the eating scenario that I visualized this morning?

REFERENCES

1. Lindsay, P.H., & Norman, D.A. (1977). *Human Information Processing: An Introduction to Psychology* (2nd ed.). New York: Academic Press.
2. Assael, H. (1995). *Consumer Behavior and Marketing Action* (5th ed.). Cincinnati, OH: South-Western College Publishing.
3. Broadbent, D. (1958). *Perception and Communication.* London, UK: Pergamon Press.
4. Sherif, M., & Cantril, H. (1945). The psychology of "attitudes": Part I. *Psychological Review, 52,* 295–319.
5. Allport, D.A. (1987). Selection for action: Some behavioural and neuro-physiological considerations of attention and action. In H. Heuer & F. Sanders (Eds.), *Perspectives on Perception and Action.* Hillsdale, NJ: Erlbaum.
6. Neumann, O. (1987). Beyond capacity: A functional view of attention. In H. Heuer & A.F. Sanders (Eds.), *Perspectives on Perception and Action* (pp. 361–394). Hillsdale, NJ: Erlbaum.
7. Van der Heijden, A.H.C. (1992). *Selective Attention and Vision.* London, UK: Routledge.
8. Wedell, D.H., Parducci, A., & Geiselman, R.E. (1987). A formal analysis of ratings of physical attractiveness: Successive contrast and simultaneous assimilation. *Journal of Experimental Social Psychology, 23,* 230–249.
9. Isaac, A.R. (1992). Mental practice—does it work in the field? *Sport Psychologist, 6,* 192–198.
10. Roure, R., Collet, C., Deschaumes-Molinaro, C., Dittmar, A., Rada H., Delhome, G., et al. (1998). Autonomic nervous system responses correlate with mental rehearsal in volleyball training. *European Journal of Applied Physiology, 78,* 99–108.
11. Porter, K., & Foster, J. (1990). *Visual Athletics.* Dubuque, IA: Wm. C. Brown Publishers.
12. Martin, K.A., & Hall, C.R. (1995). Using mental imagery to enhance intrinsic motivation. *Journal of Sport and Exercise Psychology, 17*(1), 54–69.
13. Curhan, R. (1974). The effect of merchandising and temporary promotional activities on the sales of fresh fruits and vegetables in supermarkets. *Journal of Marketing Research, 11*(3), 286–294.
14. Wilkinson, J.B., Mason, J.B., & Paksoy, C.H. (1982). Assessing the impact of short-term supermarket strategy variables. *Journal of Marketing Research, 19*(1), 72–86.
15. Frank, R.E., & Massey, W.F. (1970). Shelf position and space effects on sales. *Journal of Marking Research, 7,* 59–66.
16. Wansink, B., Painter, J.E., & Lee, Y.K. (2006). The office candy dish: Proximity's influence on estimated and actual consumption. *International Journal of Obesity, 30*(5), 871–875.

17. Assael, H. (1995). *Consumer Behavior and Marketing Action.* (5th ed.). Cincinnati, Ohio: South Western Press.
18. Neilsen, J.M., & Popkin, B.M. (2003). Patterns and trends food portion sizes. *Journal of the American Medical Association, 289*(4), 450–453.
19. Painter, J.E., Wansink, B., & Hieggelke, J.B. (2002). How visibility and convenience influence candy consumption. *Appetite, 38*(3), 237–238.
20. Wansink, B., & Kim, J. (2005). Bad popcorn in big buckets: Portion size can influence intake as much as taste. *Journal of Nutrition Education Behavior, 37*(5), 242–245.
21. Centers for Disease Control and Prevention. (2004). Trends in intake of energy and macronutrients—United States, 1971–2000. *Morbidity and Mortality Weekly Report, 53*(4), 80–82.
22. Schwartz, J., & Byrd-Bredbenner, C. (2006). Portion distortion: Typical portion sizes selected by young adults. *Journal of the American Dietetic Association, 106,* 1412–1418.
23. Diliberti, N., Bordi, P.L., Conklin, M.T., Roe, L.S., & Rolls, B.J. (2004). Increased portion size leads to increased energy intake in a restaurant meal. *Obesity Research, 12*(3), 562–568.
24. Levitsky, D.A., & Youn, T. (2004). The more food young adults are served, the more they overeat. *Journal of Nutrition, 34*(10), 2546–2549.
25. Rolls, B.J., Morris, E.L., & Roe, L.S. (2002). Portion size of food affects energy intake in normal-weight and overweight men and women. *American Journal of Clinical Nutrition, 76*(6), 1207–1213.
26. Diliberti, N., Bordi, P.L., Conklin, M.T., Roe, L.S., & Rolls, B.J. (2004). Increased portion size leads to increased energy intake in a restaurant meal. *Obesity Research, 12*(3), 562–568.
27. Rolls, B.J., Roe, L.S., Kral, T.V., Meengs, J.S., & Wall, D.E. (2004). Increasing the portion size of a packaged snack increases energy intake in men and women. *Appetite, 42*(1), 63–69.
28. Wansink, B. & Cheney, M.M. (2005). Super bowls: Serving bowl size and food consumption, *Journal of the American Medical Association, 293*(14), 1727–1728.
29. U.S. Department of Agriculture. (2005). *Dietary Guidelines for Americans, 2005.* Washington, DC: U.S. Department of Health and Human Services.
30. Young, L.R., & Nestle, M. (2002). The contribution of expanding portion sizes to the U.S. obesity epidemic. *American Journal of Public Health, 92,* 246–249.
31. Schlosser, E. (2002) *Fast Food Nation.* New York, NY: Penguin Books.

Chapter 6

Self-Perception and Eating Patterns

LEARNING OBJECTIVES

By the end of this chapter, the reader will be able to:

1. Understand how the perception of oneself can affect adherence to an eating plan.

2. Identify biases in the self-perception process that can cause incorrect diagnosis of the causes of one's eating behaviors.

3. Distinguish the difference between "downward" and "upward" comparisons that we naturally make about ourselves in relation to others' eating behavior.

4. Apply strategies that will counteract dysfunctional perceptions in order to facilitate adherence to an eating plan.

"Oh, I Am Not Like Those [Poor] Other People

Seeing yourself as better off than others or making what is called a "downward social comparison" has been shown to have many beneficial effects on health outcomes, especially with regard to adherence programs designed to get smokers to permanently quit lighting up. Gerrard and associates' 2005 study at the University of Iowa with male and female smokers who had been lighting up for over 23 years proved just that.[1]

One-hundred and fifty-one heavy smokers were asked to provide adjectives to describe the "prototypical heavy smoker." Next, these individuals were asked to give a description of their own personality characteristics. Those smokers who provided "unfavorable" prototypes of the typical heavy smoker and perceived themselves as very different from these prototypes were the individuals who were most successful in adhering to the smoking cessation program, 6 and 12 months later.

The implications from this and related studies are far reaching for all types of health and goal-oriented outcomes (e.g., survivor rate of breast cancer patients).[2,3] Make a downward social comparison, feel the motivation surge, and achieve your goal!

THE SELF-CONCEPT

Our self-concept is comprised of fairly permanent self-assessments, with regard to our personality attributes, knowledge, skills, abilities, occupation, hobbies, and awareness of our physical attributes.[4] For example, the statement "I am a hard worker" is a self-assessment that contributes to one's self-concept. In contrast, the statement "I am worn out" would not normally be considered part of someone's self-concept, since being tired is a temporary state. Regardless, a person's self-concept may change with time and is subject to reevaluation by that individual.

It is important to note that the self-concept is not restricted to the present. It typically includes past selves and future selves. Future selves or "possible selves" represent individuals' ideas of what they might become, what they would like to become, and what they are scared of becoming.[5] In other words, possible selves are made up of our hopes, fears, standards, goals, and threats. Possible selves are a great incentive for future behavior and they also provide an evaluative context for the current view of oneself.

THE DEVELOPMENT AND CHANGE OF THE SELF-CONCEPT

No one is born with a self-concept. Our self-concept gradually develops in the early years of life and is reshaped through repeated perceived experiences, particularly with significant others. Our self-concept is learned through social development and does not seem to be instinctive. Because our self-concept is based on our perceptions, individuals may perceive themselves differently from the ways others see them.

We perceive any experience that is not consistent with one's self-concept as a threat. When a person is unable to get rid of perceived inconsistencies, emotional problems can develop. Negative interpretations of oneself seem to develop when we overgeneralize and make sweeping conclusions based on little information. Additionally, these negative assessments of oneself can be created from dichotomous reasoning, which is dividing everything in terms of extremes or opposites.

Self-concepts can be resistant to change, especially when a particular belief is central to the core of one's being. At the heart of change is one's perception of potential success and failure. For instance, failure in a strongly regarded area lowers evaluations in all other areas as well. Success in a highly regarded area raises evaluations in other seemingly unrelated areas. As we can see, one's self-concept is a very dynamic and malleable structure. Consequently, the world and its happenings are not just perceived, they are perceived in relation to one's self-concept. For individuals who have a healthy self-concept, there is constant assimilation of new ideas and expulsion of old ideas throughout life. However, individuals innately strive to behave in ways that are consistent with their self-concepts, even if these behaviors are beneficial or hurtful to the self or others. Self-concept continuously guards itself against loss of self-esteem (which is one's overall assessment of personal worth), because it is this loss that produces feelings of anxiety. When one's self-concept must constantly defend itself from assault, growth opportunities for that individual are far and few between.

Self-Perception Theory

There are some aspects about our self-concept that occasionally may be unclear. For instance, sometimes our attitude toward a specific issue may be ambiguous and not part of our self-concept at that moment. It is during these ambiguous times that researcher Daryl Bem states that we look to our behaviors as a clue to that missing part of our self-concept or attitude.[6] This idea is known as the *self-perception theory*. For instance, if you want to know if "you are a healthy eater," you then look to your behavior to infer your attitude. If you are constantly indulging in fast food, you would then incorporate an attitude about yourself "I am not a healthy eater" into your self-concept. This self-assessment would no doubt affect an individual's future behavior.

Social Comparison Theory

A related theory that further accounts for how our self-concepts are altered is the *social comparison theory*.[7] This theory posits that individuals have a drive to look to others to evaluate their own opinions and abilities. People tend to compare themselves to others when they are unable to evaluate their opinions and abilities on their own.[8] For instance, a woman may know that she can run a mile in under 5 minutes. However, she cannot know if this is a good time until she compares her time with other people's times.

Leon Festinger stated that people receive better information when they compare themselves to similar, rather than dissimilar, people. Later research on the topic developed two types of social comparisons: an upward and a downward comparison. An *upward comparison* occurs when an individual compares him- or herself to someone who is better off.[9] An example of an upward comparison would be an amateur swimmer comparing her lap times to those of an Olympic swimmer. Interestingly people prefer making upward rather than downward comparisons.[10] A *downward comparison* happens when an individual compares him- or herself to someone who is worse off.[11] An example of a downward comparison would be comparing one's grade on an assignment to other students in the class who received lower grades. This form of comparison typically makes one feel good about themselves.[12] Typically, people with low self-esteem are more likely to make downward comparisons.[13] For instance, patients, who had the threat of breast cancer, coped better with it when they compared their cases with those of people who had more severe cases.[14] The information that we cull from these daily comparisons is then incorporated into our self-concept.

Attribution Theory

Our self-concept instigates many of our daily behaviors. However, once we engage in a behavior, an additional perception process occurs: the process of attribution. Many researchers believe that human beings are naïve scientists and always looking for the causes of their own behavior and the behavior of others.[15] By understanding what causes another individual's behavior or our own behavior, we are able to predict what we or others will do in the future, leaving fewer uncertainties in life. This process of ascribing a cause to a behavior is termed an *attribution*. Generally, there are two types of attributions that we make: internal and external. *Internal attributions* attribute one's behavior to dispositional causes or origins ("Frederick ate the cake because he has no willpower"). *External attributions* attribute one's behavior to situational factors ("Frederick ate the cake because it was his 30th birthday party").

Errors in the Attribution Process

We make some common errors during the attribution process that can affect the accuracy of our perceptions of our own and others' behavior. One prominent error is termed the fundamental attribution error (FAE).[16] This error is the tendency to overattribute causes of others' behavior to dispositional factors or determinants and underestimate the effects of situational factors in producing one's behavior. For instance, consistent with the FAE, if the motorist in front of you were to suddenly slam on the brakes, causing you to rear-end their car, you would immediately make an internal attribution and attribute their behavior to being a "careless driver." According to the FAE, it takes too much mental effort to search for situational clues or causes to that individual's reckless behavior (e.g., a deer ran in front of the motorist's car and that is why he slammed on the brakes) and it is easier to attribute the blame to what is prominent stimuli on our perceptual horizon, the motorist.

Another error is termed the actor-observer bias.[17] This bias is the tendency to attribute our own negative behaviors to situational factors and negative behaviors of others to their dispositions or personality attributes. The researchers theorize that this error is due to the perceiver's visual perception. When we are looking for the cause of our behavior, the prominent stimulus on our horizon is, of course, the situation before us. However, when ascribing the cause of another's behavior, the prominent stimulus on our visual horizon is that person, thus making us more likely to attribute their behavior to their personality attributes.

A related error to the actor-observer bias, is the self-serving bias.[18] This perceptual error helps to maintain an individual's self-esteem even when negative events occur in one's life. The self-serving bias occurs when an individual experiences a failure and attributes it to a situational factor beyond his or her control. For example, Rosemarie was successful at losing 50 pounds by changing her diet and regularly exercising, however, when her mother died, she regained 45 pounds. She is able to maintain her self-esteem (even though she failed in keeping the weight off) because her mother's death was a situational factor beyond her control.

Likewise, when we experience success in life, we attribute it to our internal factors. In other words, we take credit for our successes and blame our failures on others or the situation. For instance, if we receive a failing grade on a paper assignment, we would instinctively attribute it to situational factors (e.g., "the professor graded unfairly" or "I received that grade because the professor does not like me"). Likewise, if we received the highest grade in the class on our paper assignment, we would attribute it to our dispositional factors (e.g., "I put a lot of effort into that paper" or "I am a natural-born writer"). In regards to eating behaviors, if we are struggling with following our eating plan, we may blame it on situational factors such as "my job is requiring me to work extra hours and I'm too tired to cook" or "my husband insists that we keep ice cream in the house." If, however, we are successful in following our eating plan, we attribute it to our hard work and effort (e.g., "I wake up extra early every morning and make a healthy breakfast" or "I gave up my mid-afternoon cookie break at work"). Though the self-serving bias helps to maintain an individual's self-esteem level, it can prove detrimental to the individual's self-concept in the long run. Consider an individual who consistently attributes her failures to situational factors outside of her control. After many repeated situational attributions, the individual will likely develop a feeling of "learned helplessness" and feel as if her environment is uncontrollable.[19] This feeling of loss of control will prompt an individual to stop trying. People who are chronic dieters usually reach this point after many unsuccessful attempts at weight loss or weight management.

The last attributional bias that we will be discussing is termed the Pygmalion effect or self-fulfilling prophecy. This effect occurs when a person has a known expectation of another individual's behavior, thus causing that individual to behave in ways consistent with the other's expectation of him or her. This process can just as easily work for perceptions that we hold about ourselves. If we hold the belief that we have very little self-control when confronted with sweets, we will be more likely to self-fulfill this belief by acting consistent with it and indulging in sweets when they are present. The Pygmalion effect can also have positive results. A study conducted by Rosenthal in 1968 shows the upside to the self-fulfilling prophecy effect.[20] In this Oak School experiment, teachers were led to believe that specific students (who were actually chosen at random) would likely show signs of an intellectual growth spurt during the year. At the end of the academic year, the students whom the teachers expected to grow intellectually did indeed! After being assessed through an IQ test, the students in the experimental group had significantly greater gains in intellectual growth than did those in the control group. Rosenthal believes that the teachers' expectations of the students' behavior were the indirect cause of the targeted students' IQ growth. The teachers unconsciously treated these students differently than those students not expected to have an intellectual growth spurt. The teachers called on these targeted students more in class and gave additional learning reinforcement to these students. Rosenthal and Fade found the Pygmalion effect to occur in the animal kingdom as well.[21] Researchers working with laboratory rats were falsely told that one group of rats was slower and less capable than the other group of rats. Indeed at the end of the study, the experimenters' expectations of the rats' performance was fulfilled.

APPLICATION OF THE SELF-PERCEPTION PROCESS TO NUTRITION ADHERENCE

In the following part of the chapter, we will discuss how expectations about eating behavior can be positively and negatively brought to fruition. We engage in eating behavior several times a day, but fail to realize how our perceptions of ourselves can affect how much, when and what we eat.

And many times our self-perceptions are based on comparisons to others' eating behavior. These comparisons can either positively or negatively affect our eating behavior as we will soon see.

Self-Concept and Eating Behavior

One's self-concept is made up of several selves, such as the actual self, the ideal self, and the future self. These identities are based upon our past and current experiences. The good news is that one's self-concept is very malleable and can be easily changed if one is motivated to reassess it. However, individuals who have narrowly defined self-concepts and limited self-schemas (the beliefs and ideas that people have about themselves) are likely to have difficulty adhering to a desired healthy eating plan. It is important for all individuals to have a multifaceted self-schema that is rich in positive traits, while realistically incorporating one's temporary limitations. One's self-schema should ideally incorporate many realms such as personality traits, morals, values, intelligence, physical attributes, hobbies, work success, interpersonal relationship success, athleticism, spirituality, and volunteer pursuits. It is when one defines oneself on only one dimension—and defines themselves poorly on it—that it leads to low self-esteem and a higher likelihood that emotional problems will develop within, making adherence to any type of eating plan difficult. Research has revealed that this phenomenon is especially prevalent for young girls who utilize their physical bodies as their only means of self-definition.[22] In other words, girls disregard their personalities, their morals and values, and their intelligence and instead focus only on their physical appearance as the source of their identity. Thus, the body becomes of the utmost importance, the concrete notion of self, and making it beautiful and perfect is the girl's primary priority. When these unrealistic expectations are not met, emotional problems such as anxiety, depression, and disordered eating are likely to develop.[23]

A study conducted by Stein and Nyquist illustrates the relationship between negative, limited self-schemas and the development of eating disorders.[24] Their study consisted of 79 women who were previously diagnosed with an eating disorder (ED) and 34 women with no known history of an ED. The women were given a stack of 52 blank index cards and asked to write down all descriptors that were important to how they thought about themselves. Next, they were asked to rate each descriptor according to: (1) degree of self-descriptiveness, (2) degree of importance to one's self-description, and (3) whether the descriptor was positive, negative, or neutral. In keeping with previous research on self-schemas,[25] descriptors that were rated highly self-descriptive and highly important (8 to 11 on an 11-point scale) were identified as self-schemas. The number of positive self-schemas was computed by totaling the number of self-descriptors that met the criteria for a self-schema and were rated positive. The same method was used to compute the number of negative self-schemas. The results revealed that the ED group had fewer positive schemas compared to women in the control group. Also as predicted, women in the ED group demonstrated a pattern of information processing suggesting that they have a "fat" schema available in memory. Controlling for the effects of BMI and general information-processing differences, the ED group endorsed as self-descriptive a greater proportion of fat adjectives and were slower to make "not me" judgments of fat adjectives compared to the control group. When considering that all but six women in the group were currently within a low normal-to-normal weight range (BMI: mean = 22.2, range 18.2–27.9), these results support the hypothesis that women with ED have an unrealistic conception of the self as fat. The results of this study provide evidence to support the view that the relative absence of a rich and diverse collection of positive self-schemas contributes to disordered eating attitudes and behaviors. An intervention that addresses the relative deficit of positive self-schemas and the presence of more negative self-schemas should be applied.

Negative Self-Schemas of Eating Behavior

An initial assessment of self-schemas (positive and negative) of any individual who wants to adhere to a specific eating plan is a necessary step before commencing an eating plan. A method similar to the one executed in Stein and Nyquist's study can be used. Negative self-schemas with regard to physical appearance, eating behavior, self-control, and motivation should be targeted. The root of these negative self-schemas probably from a past "self", a self-concept that we held in years past, should be explored with a dietitian or counselor. Evidence should be elicited by the counselor from the client to prompt them to reassess past self-concepts and invalidate these negative self-schemas. At the same time, the counselor should explore the client's positive self-schemas and possibly draw forth more enriching adjectives from the client to build on these already existing positive schemas and create a more extensive network. Positive "future" selves should be developed as a point of reference for the client to attain.

The changing of negative self-schemas is necessary when we consider these negative schemas in the context of the Pygmalion effect. Recall that the Pygmalion effect centers around the idea that if you internalize a thought or attitude, you are more likely to bring about behaviors that are consistent with that thought in your daily interactions.

Suppose you hold a negative self-schema of yourself as lacking self-control when you are in the presence of desserts (e.g., cookies, cakes, ice cream).

When you encounter a setting with desserts present, the Pygmalion effect predicts that you will engage in behavior that is consistent with the beliefs that you hold about yourself. In this scenario, one will readily partake in eating the sweet treats, thus fulfilling one's own self-schema. Therefore, it is critical that one change any negative self-schemas that exist related to eating behavior or self-control or adherence to an eating plan will be never be achieved. In this example, a person could change their negative self-schema into a positive self-schema by internalizing the thought that they can exhibit control by taking a small amount of dessert or by politely declining an offer of dessert. In doing this, it is more likely that they will follow through with these behaviors upon their next encounter with desserts.

The Development of Negative Self-Schemas of Eating Behavior

Many negative self-schemas related to eating are developed through vicarious experiences via fashion and fitness magazines. A study by Vaughan and Fouts examined girls between 9 and 14 years old across a 16-month period.[26] The researchers found that girls who significantly increased their fashion magazine reading had an increase in ED symptoms and vice versa. In recent years, women's body sizes have grown larger, while societal standards of body shape have become much thinner.[27] This discrepancy has made it increasingly difficult for most women to achieve the current sociocultural "ideal." Such a standard of perfection is unrealistic and even dangerous. Many of the models shown in advertisements, and in other forms of popular media, are approximately 20 percent below ideal body weight, thus meeting the diagnostic criteria for anorexia nervosa.[28] Research has repeatedly shown that constant exposure to thin models causes women to develop negative body image self-schemas, leading to disordered eating in many females. Almost all forms of the media contain unrealistic images, and the negative effects of such idealistic portrayals have been demonstrated in numerous studies.[29] Findings of one study indicate that 83 percent of teenage girls reported reading fashion magazines for about 4.3 hours each week.[30] Females' motivations for reading such material varies, but self-report inventories have shown that most women who read fashion magazines do so to get information about beauty, fitness, grooming, and style.[31]

Social Comparison and Eating Behavior

Another avenue through which negative self-schemas are developed is through social comparisons. The social comparison theory offers an explanation for how media images actually impact a woman's self-schema in relation to her body and eating behavior. The social comparison theory examines how individuals evaluate themselves in relation to peers and social categories.[32] Depending on the target of comparison, a person will usually judge themselves as being either better or worse on some dimension. Recall that an upward comparison occurs when an individual compares him- or herself to someone who fares better than they do on a particular construct, whereas a downward comparisons involve a person comparing him- or herself to someone who is not as well off as they are in a certain dimension. Upward comparisons have been found to correlate with depression of mood, whereas downward comparisons are more likely to elicit elevation of mood.[33,34] Mass media seems to be one of the prominent sources to which individuals look for social comparisons. Television and advertisements in magazines provide a plethora of references for upward social comparisons. Images in the media generally project a standard to which women are expected to aspire, yet that standard is almost completely impossible for most women to achieve.

Women who report higher levels of social comparison are at greater risk to develop extreme preoccupation with weight and appearance, and are also more likely to display disordered eating patterns. This finding suggests that programs aimed at decreasing females' levels of social comparison may have some efficacy. Women who are taught not to compare themselves to unrealistic standards and be critical of images they see in the media are less likely to internalize this negative unattainable standard into their self-schemas. Several programs with such goals have been researched, and evidence has shown that such interventions seem to hold a great deal of promise.[35]

While the media's portrayal of women is not likely to change anytime soon, there is hope for altering women's internalized ideal body to reflect something that is attainable and realistic. If women can learn not to internalize the sociocultural ideal, they may be able to ward against negative body self-schemas and developing eating disorders.[36] One aspect in interventions like these is to have women made aware of the prevalence of techniques such as airbrushing and the use of such computer programs as Photoshop that photographers and advertisers use to produce these so-called idealistic images of women. With this information in hand, making an upward comparison to a media image will seem pointless to the perceiver. Additionally, these type of interventions encourage women to make downward social comparisons to similar others (e.g., with regard to age and height). This form of comparison further enhances one's self-esteem and self-schema with regard to eating behavior and body image. The person is encouraged to notice similar others who appear "farther from their dietary goals" than themselves. This form of downward comparison can be done while walking down the street or even while passing a fast food restaurant and watching someone else eat a meal not on their "healthy" eating plan. Downward comparisons generally result in motivating the evaluator and adding to that individual's network of positive body and eating self-schemas.

Attributions of Eating Behavior

Why do we eat the things that we do? This is a question that we all ask ourselves at several points in our lives. In our attempt to answer this question, we use the process of attribution, which is ascribing a cause to our behavior. Recall that we typically make either an internal attribution (e.g., attributing it to our internal characteristics) or an external attribution (e.g., attributing it to the situation). A basic rule of thumb is this: We like any of the behaviors that we have freely chosen to engage in; those behaviors that we are forced to engage in, we like less. Additionally, when there is an external reason (or sufficient justification) as to why we do a certain behavior, then we attribute that as the cause of our behavior. For instance, suppose that we drink club soda because it helps to soothe our upset stomach. When we question why we drink club soda, we will most likely attribute it to the fact that it soothes our stomach, not to our fondness of it. However, if we can find no external cause for our behavior, we assume that we did the behavior because we liked it and that is who we are. When we make an internal attribution for our behavior, we are more likely to engage in that behavior in the future. Conversely, if we see our behavior as externally motivated, then we are less likely to freely engage in that behavior in the future. So, with regard to the domain of nutrition adherence, one would want to foster eating adherence behaviors that are internally motivated because they will have a higher likelihood of being repeated in the future.

Suppose one's eating plan prescribed by a dietitian includes eating a high-fiber breakfast cereal on a regular basis. Because eating this type of food(s) is externally motivated (prescribed by the dietitian), typically one would attribute their eating behavior to this external source and the likelihood of this client adhering to this eating plan would be low. However, if the client made an internal attribution for his or her eating behavior ("I really like the taste of this high-fiber breakfast cereal and that is why I eat it"), then he or she would be more likely to adhere to eating the high-fiber cereal in the future. In other words, persons who are intrinsically motivated to perform a certain behavior will be more likely to sustain that behavior in the long run, than those individuals who are extrinsically motivated. The take-home message then is that individuals should be encouraged to make internal attributions for their positive eating behaviors, even if these behaviors are originally instigated by an external factor or person (e.g., physician, dietitian).

Attributions can also explain other roadblocks that we might encounter when trying to adhere to a specific eating plan. The self-serving bias and the actor-observer bias are two of these roadblocks of which to be aware. These biases occur when we attribute negative behaviors in our lives to situational causes and positive behaviors to internal factors. When these biases occur in the context of our eating behavior, we can see the many negative implications. Suppose Trisha's eating plan stipulates for her to eat 1,500 calories a day. For several days Trisha successfully adheres to this goal and naturally attributes her success internally to her strong willpower. However, on the fourth day of her eating plan, things go awry and Trish ends up consuming 1,000 more calories than stipulated by her eating plan. Being consistent with the self-serving bias and actor-observer bias, Trisha attributes her noncompliance to an external factor, her boss who made her stay late at work to finish up a project and this disrupted her daily eating schedule. While an external factor may indeed have contributed to part of the problem, if Trisha continues to attribute her adherence failure to external circumstances beyond her control, her eating behavior will spiral downward. This continued pattern of externalizing failures will induce a sense of "learned helplessness" in Trisha. She will come to learn that much of her eating behavior is situational and out of her control, prompting inaction on her part. The learned helplessness theory posits that when we believe that we cannot control our own environment, we stop responding to it and let it take control. Therefore, one can see the potential problems that arise out of the actor-observer bias and the self-serving bias within the domain of eating adherence.

How can one ensure that these perceptual biases do not stymie one's attempts at adherence behavior? Realistically evaluating the role of situational eating factors is the key to not letting these biases put a halt to adherence efforts. Consider Juan, who attributes his nonadherence to his eating plan due to a thyroid condition. Indeed, this may be an external contributing factor, but Juan should be making an internal attribution as well for not seeking professional help to rectify his thyroid condition. When Juan attributes his nonadherence behavior in this manner, a pattern of learned helplessness will be unlikely to develop because Juan will perceive that he has control over the situational factor leading to his noncompliance. This sense of perceived control will motivate Juan to take action to control his eating environments. In summary, one should never make an external attribution alone for one's noncompliance to an eating plan, but search for a related internal factor to account for the behavior as well. These paired attributions will foster a sense of self-efficacy in the target individual for shaping a proactive eating environment in which they will thrive.

You Diagnose It

ADHERENCE SCENARIO 1

Anita has told her dietitian that she is about to give up on her eating plan of omitting red meat from her diet. These are some of the comments that Anita has relayed to her dietitian:

"It seems as if my family is always trying to thwart my efforts toward my eating plan."

"My husband will bring home fast food hamburgers for dinner or I find out that my children's soccer awards banquet is being held at a steakhouse."

1. Discuss two perceptual errors that Anita is making to account for her noncompliance to her eating plan.
2. Outline two methods by which Anita could correct these perceptual errors and gain more control over her eating environment.

ADHERENCE SCENARIO 2

Kasey is talking with his counselor who has just urged him to make a radical change in his eating behavior. Kasey shrugs his shoulders and says, "I just don't think that I can do it. This is the way I have always eaten. It is just part of who I am."

1. Discuss the prominent perceptual stumbling block to change that Kasey is facing.
2. As a counselor, lay out a plan that focuses on altering perceptions to eliminate Kasey's resistance to a new eating plan.

Review

✓ Our self-concept is comprised of fairly permanent self-assessments, such our personality attributes, knowledge of our skills and abilities, our occupation and hobbies, and awareness of our physical attributes.

✓ No one is born with a self-concept. Our self-concept develops gradually in the early years of life and is reshaped through repeated perceived experiences, particularly with significant others.

✓ Festinger's social comparison theory (1954) posits that individuals have a drive to look to others to evaluate their own opinions and abilities. People tend to compare themselves to others when they are unable to evaluate their opinions and abilities on their own.

✓ This process of ascribing a cause to a behavior is termed an attribution. Generally, there two types of attributions that we make: internal and external. Internal attributions attribute one's behavior to dispositional causes or origins. External attributions attribute one's behavior to situational factors.

✓ The self-serving bias occurs when an individual experiences a failure and attributes it to a situational factor beyond his or her control.

D.I.E.T. (Do I Eat This?)

TIPS TO CONSIDER WHEN REACHING FOR A PIECE OF FOOD

- Is my self-concept consistent with eating this type of food?
- Is my decision to eat this food due to the expectations of others present at the table?
- Am I reaching for this piece of food because everyone else is doing it?
- Would someone on a similar eating plan, but who lacks my motivation and willpower, eat this?

REFERENCES

1. Gerrard, M., Lane, D.J., & Stock, M.L. (2005). Smoking cessation: Social comparison level predicts success for adult smokers. *Health Psychology, 24*, 623–629.
2. Taylor, S.E., Wood, J.V., & Lichtman, R.R. (1983). It could be worse: Selective evaluation as a response to victimization. *Journal of Social Issues, 39*(2), 19–40.
3. Gibbons, F.X., Benbow, C.P., & Gerrard, M. (1994). From top dog to bottom half: Social comparison strategies in response to poor performance. *Journal of Personality and Social Psychology, 67*, 638–652.
4. Markus, H., & Nurius, P. (1986). Possible selves. *American Psychologist, 41*, 954–969.
5. Berry, D., Oyserman, D., & Terry, K. (2006). Possible selves and academic outcomes: How and when possible selves impel action. *Journal of Personality and Social Psychology, 91*, 188–204.
6. Bem, D. (1967). Self-perception: An alternative interpretation of cognitive dissonance phenomena. *Psychological Review, 74*(3), 183–200.
7. Festinger, L. (1957). *A Theory of Cognitive Dissonance*. Stanford, CA: Stanford University Press.
8. Martin, R., Suls, J., & Wheeler, L. (2001). Psychology of social comparison. *International Encyclopedia of the Social and Behavioral Sciences*, 14254–14257.
9. Baumeister, R.F., & Bushman, R.J. (2008). *Social Psychology and Human Nature*. Stamford, CT: Thompson Learning.
10. Wills, T.A. (1981). Downward comparison principles in social psychology. *Psychological Bulletin, 90*, 245–271.

11. Baumeister, R.F., & Bushman, R.J. (2008). *Social Psychology and Human Nature.* Stamford, CT: Thompson Learning.
12. Ibid.
13. Ibid.
14. Gibbons, F.X., Gerrard, M., Lane, D.J., & Stock, M.L. (2005). Smoking cessation: Social comparison level predicts success for adult smokers. *Health Psychology, 24,* 623–629.
15. Heider, F. (1958). *The Psychology of Interpersonal Relations.* New York: John Wiley & Sons.
16. Ross, L. (1977). The intuitive psychologist and his shortcomings: Distortions in the attribution process. In L. Berkowitz (Ed.), *Advances in Experimental Social Psychology* (Vol. 10). New York: Academic Press.
17. Jones, E., & Nisbett, R. (1971). *The Actor and the Observer: Divergent Perceptions of Causes of Behavior.* New York: General Learning Press.
18. Miller, D.T., & Ross, M. (1975). Self-serving biases in the attribution of causality: Fact or fiction? *Psychological Bulletin, 82,* 213–225.
19. Hiroto, D.S., & Seligman, M.E.P. (1975). Generality of learned helplessness in man. *Journal of Personality and Social Psychology, 31,* 311–327.
20. Rosenthal, R., & Jacobson, L. (1968). *Pygmalion in the Classroom: Teacher Expectation and Pupils' Intellectual Development.* New York: Rinehart and Winston.
21. Rosenthal, R., & Fade, K.L. (1963). The effect of experimenter bias on the performance of the albino rat. *Behavioural Science, 8,* 183–189.
22. Schupak-Neuberg, E., & Nemeroff, C. (1993). Disturbances in identity and self-regulation in bulimia nervosa: Implications for a metaphorical perspective of "body as self." *International Journal Disorders, 13,* 335.
23. Fairburn, C.G., Hay, P.J., & Welch, S.L. (1993). Binge eating and bulimia nervosa: Distribution and determinants. In C.G. Fairburn & G.T. Wilson (Eds.), *Binge Eating: Nature, Assessment, and Treatment* (pp. 123–143). New York: Guilford.
24. Stein, K., & Nyquist, L. (2001), Disturbance in the self: A source of eating disorders. *Eating Disorders Review, 12*(1).
25. Kendzierski, D., & Whitaker, D. J. (1997). The role of self-schema in linking intentions with behavior. *Personality and Social Psychology Bulletin, 23,* 139–147.
26. Vaughan, K., & Fouts, G. (2003). Changes in television and magazine exposure and eating disorder symptomatology. *Sex Roles, 49*(7/8), 313–320.
27. Spitzer, B.L., Henderson, K.A., & Zivian, M.T. (1999). Gender differences in population versus media body sizes: A comparison over four decades. *Sex Roles, 40,* 545–565.
28. Dittmar, H., & Howard, S. (2004). Professional hazards? The impact of models' body size on advertising effectiveness and women's body-focused anxiety in professions that do and do not emphasize the cultural ideal of thinness. *British Journal of Social Psychology, 43*(4), 477–497.
29. Schooler, D., Ward, M., Merriwether, A., & Caruthers, A. (2004). Who's that girl: Television's role in the body image development of young white and black female. *Psychology of Female Quarterly, 28*(1), 38–47.
30. Thompson, J.K., Heinberg, L.J., Altabe, M., & Tantleff-Dunn, S. (1999). *Exacting Beauty: Theory, Assessment and Treatment of Body Image Disturbance.* Washington, DC: American Psychological Association.

31. Tiggemann, M. (2003). Media exposure, body dissatisfaction and disordered eating: Television and magazines are not the same! *European Eating Disorders Review, 11*(5), 418–430.

32. Milkie, M.A. (1999). Social comparisons, reflected appraisals, and mass media: The impact of pervasive beauty images on black and white girls' self concepts. *Social Psychology Quarterly, 62*(2), 190–210.

33. Lin, L.F., & Kulik, J.A. (2002). Social comparison and women's body satisfaction. *Basic & Applied Social Psychology, 24*(2), 115–123.

34. Schooler, D., Ward, L.M., Merriwether, A., & Caruthers, A. (2004). Who's that girl: Television's role in the body image development of young white and black women. *Psychology of Women Quarterly, 28*(1), 38–47.

35. Thompson, J.K., & Coovert, M.D. (1999). Body image, social comparison, and eating disturbance: A covariance structure modeling. *International Journal of Eating Disorders, 26*(1), 43–51.

36. Sands, E.R., & Wardle, J. (2003). Internalization of ideal body shapes in 9–12-year-old girls. *International Journal of Eating Disorders, 33*(2), 193–204.

Chapter 7

Emotion Perception and Eating Patterns

LEARNING OBJECTIVES

By the end of this chapter, the reader will be able to:

1. Identify the five stages of perceiving an emotion.
2. Distinguish between emotional hunger and physical hunger.
3. Identify environmental triggers of emotion-based eating.
4. Apply strategies that will weaken the association between emotions and food to facilitate adherence to an eating plan.

Emotion-Based Eating

"That was such a sad movie. I cried during the whole thing . . . oh, and can you pass me the popcorn?"

This might have been a common sentiment and behavior of many of the 30 participants in Garg, Wansink, and Inman's 2007 study after watching the movie *Love Story*.[1] Yes, Garg and colleagues compensated their participants for watching two movies by providing them with hot, buttery popcorn during the screenings.

The researchers were able to successfully induce emotional states within their participants by having them watch two types of movies: the sad movie *Love Story*, and the happy movie *Sweet Home Alabama*. While watching the movies, the participants were given large buckets of hot, buttery popcorn.

As theorized, when watching the sad movie, the participants consumed 28 percent more popcorn than when watching the happy movie. Through several related studies, the researchers concluded that people tend to eat more hedonic, or pleasant tasting, food, such as M&Ms and popcorn, when they are in a sad state and less hedonic food, such as raisins, when they are in a happy state.

With this knowledge in hand, no doubt movie theater food concession stands are stocked up with hedonistic foods to satisfy moviegoers' cravings that result from all types of movies.

EXPERIENCING AN EMOTION

An *emotion* is a mental and physiological state that is connected with a wide array of feelings, thoughts, and behaviors. How and when one experiences an emotion is different for every person because emotions are subjective experiences. The basic sequential stages of experiencing an emotion typically are appraisal, physical response, facial expressions, nonverbal behavior, and motives[2] (see **Figure 7–1**), though some researchers argue that the order differs slightly.[3,4]

The following is an example to further illustrate the process of experiencing an emotion:

> Tina receives an acceptance letter in the mail to her number one college choice. First, Tina perceives/appraises the stimuli that something fantastic has happened. Next, Tina exhibits the relevant physical behavioral response to this emotion such as jumping up and down; her pulse will probably quicken as well. Her facial expressions will reveal a smile and she will engage in nonverbal behavior such as giving a victory sign with her hand. The last stage that she will engage in is the motivation to tell others of her joy and acceptance letter.

It is important to realize, as other researchers such as Lazarus and Zajonc have put forth that the steps of experiencing emotion can occur out of order and do not have to each occur separately. For instance, the James-Lange Theory posits that emotional experience is largely due to the experience of bodily changes.[5,6] An example would be that after contracting the stomach flu, one would experience the emotion of feeling miserable. The functionalist approach, on the other hand, posits that emotions have evolved for a particular function, such as to keep the subject safe.[7] This approach indicates that individuals experience the motive first (such as keeping one's young out of harm's way) and then the emotions (e.g., anger, alarm) follow. Regardless, one should take away the understanding that experiencing an emotion is a complex synthesis of thoughts, physical sensations, and motivations.

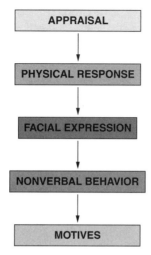

Figure 7–1 The Stages of Perceiving an Emotion.

Also, keep in mind that emotions generally arise from three different sources. The most obvious source of emotions is from a present stimulus, such as watching a sad movie. Second, emotions can arise from classical conditioning, as mentioned in Chapter 2. For instance, if you drive by your old high school, you may automatically feel a sense of happiness, due to the fun that you experienced there. Lastly, emotions can arise from just thinking about a past experience or memory. For example, thinking back about seeing your favorite comedian perform may bring about a sense of amusement and happiness.

TYPES OF EMOTIONS

How many emotions can a human being possibly experience? No one is really sure, but it was found once that there are 17,953 terms for personality traits in the English dictionary.[8] This number can serve as a good reference point for potentially how many different types of emotions a person might be able to experience. One way to categorize the many emotions that we experience is through the emotional circumplex model. The model assumes that all emotions vary along two dimensions from aroused to unaroused and from negative to positive.[9,10] For instance in **Figure 7–2**, the emotion, "tense" is very aroused and negative, while the emotion of "gloomy" is very unaroused and negative. The emotional circumplex model is a useful method for comparing emotions to one another and understanding their roots.

Regardless of whether an emotion is positive or negative, individuals differ in the intensity that they experience an emotion as well as the rate with

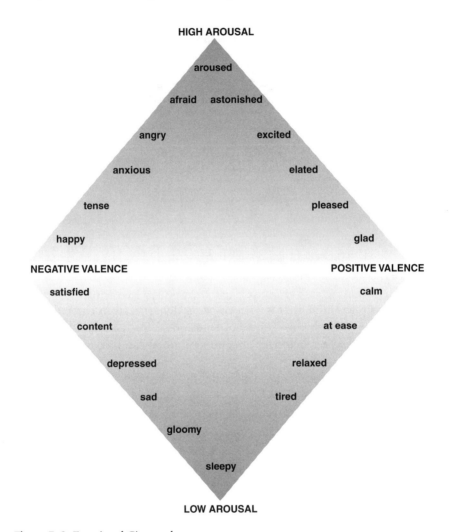

Figure 7–2 Emotional Circumplex.
Source: Adapted from Russell J.A. (1980) A circumplex model of affect. *Journal of Personality and Social Psychology,* 39:1161–1178.

which they change from one emotion to another. Research has revealed that people who are high in affect intensity (the intensity of an emotion) seem to experience emotions, especially joy and sadness, more intensely than others.[11] In addition, these intense emotions can lead to intense physiological arousal that may end up harming the heart and the immune system.[12] With regard to the rapid change of emotions, a study by Eaton and Funder had participants report their emotions fours times a day for 8 days.[13] The participants whose emotions showed the highest fluctuation of change described themselves and were described by people who knew them well as "generally fearful" and "hostile." The researchers surmise that these individuals' emotion swings cause stress for themselves and others around them, thus producing the hostile and fearful personality traits. They also conjecture that maybe these individuals lacked a solid emotional base, resulting in them being overly susceptible to being buffeted by the ever-changing landscape of life.

APPLICATION OF EMOTION PERCEPTION TO NUTRITION ADHERENCE

Emotional eating is eating for reasons other than hunger—so instead of the physical symptom of hunger initiating the eating, an emotion triggers one's eating. Emotional eating can be a conscious or unconscious consumption of sweetened, salty, or fatty foods, usually to excess. Many people, even those who are not overweight, have some sense of the connection between emotions and diet.

Food and feelings naturally go together. From birth, we have associated food with pleasantness, nurturing, and affection. Eating for comfort is a common behavior and comes from a deep association between the experience of eating and the feeling of comfort as the following quote illustrates.

> *"Chocolate is cheaper than therapy and you don't need an appointment."*
> —Unknown

A variety of psychological theories with regard to emotional eating have been developed through the years. One theory posits that emotional eating is the failure to attain the basic needs in life (e.g., safety, security).[14] Additionally, these researchers assert that when an individual perceives life situations to be stressful, they utilize their own internal resources (e.g., self-esteem, humor) and external resources (e.g., friends, family) to buffer themselves against the stress. However, if one's needs are still not met, then food consumption may be used as an additional resource to complement the deficit.

Another theory concerning the roots of emotional eating suggests that confusion and apprehension in recognizing and accurately responding to emotional states related to hunger and satiety instigate emotional eating.[15] Also, there is a composite "escape theory" of eating that Heatherton and Baumeister propose which argues that eating is an escape from oneself.[16] Heatherton and colleagues further hypothesized that distress that threatens one's self-image acts as an instigator for disinhibition.[17] When not feeling inhibited, an individual is motivated to escape from self-awareness by redirecting their attention away from unpleasant self thoughts to food cues in the environment, which is aversive when they encounter negative information about oneself. All of the research conducted in the realm of emotional eating seems to unanimously conclude that emotional eating fails to produce any true and lasting benefit to psychological and mood states, while increased or repeated emotional eating more likely fosters mood dysphoria.

MOOD STATES AND EATING BEHAVIOR

Research has found that one's food preference is changed across a range of mood states, with individuals preferring "junk food" or food that has no nutritional value when they experience negative mood states. On the other hand, when individuals experience positive mood states, they reveal a preference for healthy foods.[18,19]

There is a great deal of talk these days about comfort foods. According to Dr. Brian Wansink, director of the Food and Brand Lab at the University of Illinois, *comfort foods* are the foods a person eat to obtain or maintain a feeling. Comfort foods are often incorrectly associated with negative moods; that people eat these foods when they are down or upset. However, many times, comfort foods are eaten to maintain pleasant and positive moods. Through research, Wansink and SeaBum learned that ice cream is first on the comfort food list.[20] After ice cream, comfort foods break down by the sex of the consumer. Wansink has found that for women, chocolate and cookies are next on the list of preferences; for men, it's pizza, steak, and casseroles. More generally speaking, though, Wansink found that people in happy moods tended to prefer foods such as pizza or steak, while sad people reached for ice cream and cookies; 36 percent of bored people opened up a bag of potato chips. It is typical for all people to eat for emotional reasons sometimes. However, when eating becomes the main strategy a person uses to manage his or her emotions, that is when it becomes dysfunctional behavior. Problems arise particularly if the foods a person chooses to eat to satisfy that emotion are not healthy. One problem that can occur by eating when one is not hungry is weight gain. Because the body does not need the calories, the extra calories get stored as fat; too much fat storage can cause one to be overweight, thus inducing health risks. Many times overeating can be attributed to emotion-based eating, so developing effective solutions to deal with one's emotions is imperative. Blair, Lewis, and Booth confirmed this finding with a weight-loss study that indicated individuals who decreased their emotional eating lost significantly more weight than those who did not.[21]

Stress and Eating Behavior

Feeding one's feelings of anxiety with food is another type of emotional association. Ganley's research indicated that stress-associated eating is more prevalent in those who are overweight but the direction of the association is unclear.[22] Observation suggests that although weight gain caused by emotional eating may exacerbate negative mood states, the latter may trigger a cycle of further emotional eating and continued weight gain. Geliebter and Aversa found that overweight individuals had increased urges to eat in response to negative emotions and situations when compared to normal weight individuals.[23] Keep in mind that such associations are highly dependent on the current emotional state of the participants. For example, a study by Ruderman demonstrated that obese women ate significantly less when highly anxious than when mildly anxious.[24] These associations do not support the idea that overeating is an attempt to alleviate aversive mood states or that all obesity is the product of emotional eating or even that stress has a unilateral relationship with food consumption.

Interestingly, the natural instinct during stress is to decrease food consumption, which reflects activation of the sympathetic nervous system.[25] When the sympathetic nervous system is activated, blood is diverted away from the digestive system to other systems that are required for defense. Stone and Brownell's study supported this assertion, revealing that subjects were more likely to eat less the higher levels of stress that they experienced.[26] Although eating when stressed does not fit the previously discussed physiological model, stress is thought to disrupt restraint and postingestional satiety signals to the brain. Work by Meisel and colleagues showed a prominent increase in body weight and enlarged adrenal glands in female Syrian hamsters when socially stressed by being caged in groups compared to those housed individually.[27] As additional support of the associations between appetite and stress, animal and human studies of depression indicate a decreased responsiveness to rewards (sucrose solution) under conditions of chronic mild stress, but the opposite when the animals, with comparable neurological systems to humans, are provided with sweeter pellets.[28] The latter finding could be due to intrinsic regulatory mechanisms being compromised when concentrations of certain food components are noticeably higher than those found in nature. The high hedonic value of fat and simple carbohydrate (sugar) concentrations in many manufactured foods, including chocolate, may overstimulate positive feedback and, and jointly with the learned expectations of alleviation of aversive mood, override normal postingestive satiety feedback signals.

Carbohydrate Consumption and Its Affect on Mood State

As one can see, studying the effects on mood after ingestion of carbohydrates is confounded by a host of methodological variables. These variable can include time with regard to eating (i.e., during the stressful moment or after the stressful event has passed) if participants are cravers or noncravers of carbohydrates, and the real mood state (e.g., depression, boredom, anxiety).

Many studies have found varied results due to these methodological issues and variable confounds. In a study by Lieberman and associates, noncarbohydrate cravers and lean subjects reported an increase in sleepiness after a carbohydrate-rich snack, while obese cravers reported a marked improvement in mood.[29] In Wurtman and Wurtman's study, they found that carbohydrate consumption produced an initial temporary relief from a sense of melancholia.[30] Also, Johnson and Larson found prominent post-binge dysphoria with some occasional, though fleeting, relief of the uncomfortable mood state.[31] Thayer's research demonstrated a longer-term reaction of reduced energy, fostering a cycle that contributed to the development and maintenance of depression.[32] In Hetherington and Macdiarmid's retrospective study, they reported that any mood improvement was only during the consumption period process, with negative moods returning immediately after consumption stopped.[33] In a study of "chocolate addicts," Macdiarmid and Hetherington found that these individuals were more depressed than the control participants, and their negative mood states were not relieved after chocolate consumption.[34] They found that chocolate eating resulted in a slight increase in contentment when eating the chocolate, but the authors believed that this is due to satiety rather than an improvement in mood, because ratings of depression or feeling relaxed were unaffected.

Additional research indicates chocolate may have a stronger physiological effect than once thought. Hill and colleagues have found that negative mood states are common among chocolate cravers and cravers have an increased tendency toward emotional eating.[35] Low central nervous system levels of serotonin have been linked with depression and obsessive-compulsive disorder. Consumption of carbohydrates, especially chocolate, has been purposed to increase levels of tryptophan uptake and the production of serotonin by the brain, resulting in an improved mood and emotional state following chocolate consumption.[36]

Hill and colleagues also examined guilt after food consumption and found that resisting a craving increases an individual's positive mood.[37] Additionally, there is widespread support for the assertion that a positive mood can be attained by eliminating refined sucrose and caffeine.[38,39,40]

Despite reoccurring methodological issues, the general findings from these studies uphold the suggestion that continued ingestion of simple carbohydrates (sugar) most likely contributes to the maintenance of a dysphoric mood.

PERCEIVING PHYSICAL HUNGER VERSUS EMOTIONAL HUNGER

There are several differences between emotional hunger and physical hunger of which to be aware. Let's look at physical hunger first. Physical hunger comes on gradually and intensifies over time. Hunger signals come from your stomach and may include "growls," pangs, or hollow feelings. Some individuals even have a sensation of nausea when they are extremely hungry. Physical hunger signals also come from your brain, letting you know that your energy supply is depleted. Some of these signals may be a sense of fogginess, lack of concentration, fatigue, or a headache. It should also be mentioned that while experiencing true hunger, you will not have any cravings for a specific food, because any food will do—and when you are full, you will stop eating.

Emotional hunger, on the other hand, starts suddenly without any warning. With emotional hunger, you will have a craving for a specific food, such as pizza or ice cream, and only that food will meet your need. Interestingly, emotional hunger feels like it needs to be satisfied instantly with the food you crave, while physical hunger can wait. The craving does not intensify over time like physical hunger and if you do something else to divert your attention away from the feeling, the craving usually will disappear. Also, if you're eating to satisfy an emotional need, you're more likely to keep eating even though you are physically full. A technique commonly used to learn how to identify physical sensations relative to hunger and fullness is the Hunger/Fullness Rating Scale as illustrated in **Figure 7–3**.

To use this scale, first note what level of hunger you are currently experiencing. If you are at level 5 or above, you are not hungry and your body does not physically need food. If you are craving a food, it is emotion-based hunger, not physical. If you are at level 3 or 4, your body is telling you that it physically needs some food. This feeling will intensify over time. If you are at level 1 or 2, you are probably too hungry and your body most definitely needs food. The problem with waiting until you get to this level is that you are so hungry that when you do finally sit down to eat, you will probably overeat or you will choose to eat something that is quick and convenient but not necessarily healthy.

The optimal time to eat is at level 3 or 4. At this point, you are experiencing physical hunger, and your body is signaling to you that you need food.

10	Truly, absolutely stuffed
9	So stuffed that it hurts
8	Very full and bloated
7	Almost starting to feel uncomfortable
6	Feeling like you have overeaten a bit
5	Very comfortable
4	First signals that your body needs food
3	Strong signals to eat
2	Very irritable and hungry
1	Extreme hunger, dizziness

Figure 7–3 Hunger/Fullness Rating Scale.
Source: Adapted from The Princeton Longevity Center Medical News, (2005). *3 "Internal" Tools for Weight Control.*

You will still have enough control to choose healthy foods and control your portions. As you eat, you can also use the scale to assess your level of fullness. To do this, stop eating when you have finished half of your meal or snack and assess where you are at with your level of fullness. If you are at a 5, you should stop eating; your body is physically telling you that you have had enough. If you are unsure of your level of fullness, take several more bites of your food and then stop again to assess your level of fullness. As you practice this technique, you will find it gets easier to consume the right quantity of food to meet your body's physical need for nourishment. It will also help to identify when your body is not physically in need of food and when your "hunger" is more emotional.

EFFECTIVE SOLUTIONS FOR EMOTION-BASED HUNGER

When craving foods, it is imperative to determine whether the craving is emotion-based hunger or physical hunger. When one has discovered *why* they want to eat, then they can devise a game plan. If it is determined that the hunger is emotion based, steps can be taken to dissipate the craving in a manner other than eating the food that is craved. As just discussed, many emotional cravings have their roots in stress. Stress-reduction techniques can include taking a long hot bath, going for a walk, relaxation exercises, journaling, listening to music, or yoga. Choosing an activity that is counterproductive to eating by involving the use of your hands is another good option. Examples of this would be knitting, crocheting, scrapbooking, crafts, or any other hobby that utilizes your hands. Another alternative would be to drink a glass of water. As discussed in an upcoming chapter, feelings of thirst can sometimes mimic feelings of hunger and a glass of water may be just the solution that the body needs. Last, apply the 10-minute rule. If you are experiencing a craving, wait 10 minutes for it to subside. If the food craving does not subside, eat a small portion of the food. Having that food proportioned out in a small plastic bag, cup, or bowl will help to prevent bingeing on the food and prevent feelings of guilt as a result of bingeing.

CORRECTLY PERCEIVING MOOD STATES AND EMOTIONAL EATING

The first step one needs to take to overcome emotion-based eating is to correctly perceive the emotion one is feeling and the craving that it produces. Refer to **Figure 7–4** as an aid in determining the type of hunger that you are experiencing.

Keeping a food or feeling log like the template illustrated in **Figure 7–5** will shed light on when you are eating for emotional-induced reasons. The food/feeling log will also capture a pattern of stimuli or triggers that are instigating your emotion-based eating behavior. Through this activity of self-monitoring, you will be able to identify triggers and emotions that lead you to eat when you may not be physically hungry. You may also learn

Question to Ask Yourself	True	False
1. "I am experiencing hunger pangs in my stomach."		
2. "My stomach feels empty."		
3. "My hunger came on slowly."		
4. "I am not craving any particular kind of food."		
5. "My mind feels unclear and it is difficult to concentrate."		
Total		

Figure 7–4 Physical Hunger Versus Emotional Hunger Checklist.

Date: Tuesday

Time	Stimulus/Trigger (e.g., physical hunger, emotion, situation, motivation)	Location (where you ate the food item)	Food Item	Hunger/Fullness Level (Rate your level of hunger/fullness before eating and after eating)	Quantity	Calories
7:32 AM	Physical hunger	Kitchen table	Oatmeal with 2% milk	3 / 4	1 cup with $^1/_2$ cup milk	260
10:45 AM	Friend offered me part of his granola bar	Break room at work	Granola bar	3 / 3	$^1/_2$ bar	135
12:30 PM	Set lunch time break at work	At my desk	Turkey sandwich, white bread, no mayo, lettuce, 1 cup of chicken noodle soup	4 / 5	1 sandwich (2 bread slices) 8 oz soup	240 / 70
4:10 PM	Discovered that my car had a flat tire: frustrated and upset	After I returned from parking lot: at my desk	Chocolate Hershey Kisses	4 / 4	10	280

Figure 7–5 Sample Food Log Template.

what time of the day or night that you are more likely to overeat. Optimally, your food/feeling log should be kept for a minimum of 1 month. Choose a small notebook that is convenient to carry with you at all times. Have it handy with a pen or pencil to capture all of your eating experiences.

To improve accuracy, you should record data within 15 minutes after finishing a meal or snack. Do not wait until the end of the day to record your data. You will forget the specifics of what occurred, how much you ate, how you were feeling, the time of day, and other important information. The more accurate your data is, the easier it will be for you to identify patterns and trends, similarities in situations, timing, thoughts, emotions, and feelings. Once you have this information, you can then begin to take steps to resolve particular problem areas.

Next, you need to learn strategies other than eating to manage the emotions you are experiencing. A number of emotions that we associate with food have been learned or conditioned since childhood. For instance, when a child is sad, the parent may try to cheer them up with some type of sweet treat. This behavior will probably get reinforced year after year until we as adults practice the same behavior. Therefore, we never learn how to deal with the sad feeling because we have always masked it with a sweet treat. Learning how to deal with feelings without food is a skill that many of us have never mastered. If you review the food/feeling log template, you can see that physical hunger did not precede the consumption of the chocolate kisses. Karen rated her hunger level at a 4 before eating the chocolate and a 4 afterwards. She most likely experienced a very short, temporary feeling of relief when she was eating the chocolate, however, eating the chocolate did not "fix" her problem. She still had to deal with her flat tire after eating the chocolate. As Karen continues to keep her food/feeling log, she may begin to see that whenever she experiences strong feelings of frustration, she turns to chocolate. Once she identifies this pattern, she can then begin to brainstorm other, nonfood methods to cope with her feelings of frustration.

SOLUTIONS FOR MANAGING EMOTIONAL EATING

Here are some strategies to counter emotional eating:

- Distinguish emotional eating from physical hunger and learn what triggers this behavior in you by keeping a food/feeling log. Use the hunger/fullness scale as part of your self-monitoring. At the end of the week, look for patterns or trends in your eating behaviors, then begin to make changes to curtail emotional eating.

- Make a list of things to do when you get the urge to eat and you're not physically hungry. Carry this list with you and put another copy of it on your refrigerator or pantry door. When you feel emotionally overwhelmed and are ready to reach for food, delay the desire by doing an enjoyable activity from your list. In essence, you are developing an association between a particular emotion and an enjoyable activity (other than eating).

- Try taking a walk, calling a friend, playing cards, cleaning your room, doing laundry, or something else, such as taking a nap, that will shift your mindset.

- Develop a new comfort food that is healthy. Try a steaming cup of herbal tea, a baked potato with salsa, or a cup of fresh fruit in a pretty parfait glass. Comfort foods do not need to be unhealthy foods.

- Sometimes it is very difficult to unlearn the association between a mood and a particular food. In that case, eat a *small portion* of the food; learning moderation is the key.

- Wansink reminds us that our memory of a food peaks after about four bites, so if you only have four bites, a few days later, you will recall the food as just as enjoyable as if you ate the entire helping.[41] In other words, if you eat just a few bites of the leftover birthday cake, you will rate eating bites of the cake just as pleasurable as if you ate the entire remaining cake—all without the cost of excess calories and sugar.

You Diagnose It

ADHERENCE SCENARIO 1

Eliza notes in her food/feeling log that she overeats throughout the day on Tuesdays and Thursdays. She is aware that her regional manager, who can be very demanding and who works in her branch office on those days, may be related to her overeating.

1. What strategies could Eliza apply on Tuesdays and Thursdays that would help to thwart her overeating tendencies?

2. Develop a long-range plan for Eliza so that she will no longer associate her regional manager with food and overeating.

ADHERENCE SCENARIO 2

Miguel works as a server at Steve's Steakhouse. Since working for the past year, Miguel has gained 23 pounds. Miguel thinks that the quick pace of the job makes him hungrier than usual.

1. What would be another alternative explanation to Miguel's overeating?
2. By using the stages of the perception of emotion process, develop a plausible order to the perception process that would explain Miguel's emotion-based eating.

Review

✓ An emotion is a mental and physiological state that is connected with a wide array of feelings, thoughts, and behaviors.

✓ The basic sequential stages of experiencing an emotion typically are appraisal, physical response, facial expressions, nonverbal behavior, and motives.

✓ The James-Lange theory posits that emotional experience is largely due to the experience of bodily changes.

✓ The functionalist approach, on the other hand, posits that emotions have evolved for a particular function, such as to keep the subject safe.

✓ The emotional circumplex model assumes that all emotions vary along two dimensions: from aroused to unaroused and from negative to positive.

✓ Comfort foods are foods that a person eats to obtain or maintain a feeling.

✓ General findings with regard to emotion-based eating uphold the suggestion that continued ingestion of simple carbohydrates most likely contributes to the maintenance of a dysphoric mood.

✓ Emotional hunger starts suddenly without any warning. With emotional hunger, you will have a craving for a specific food, such as pizza or ice cream, and only that food will meet your need.

✓ Physical hunger comes on gradually and will intensify over time. Hunger signals come from your stomach and may include growls, pangs, or hollow feelings.

D.I.E.T. (Do I Eat This?)

TIPS TO CONSIDER WHEN REACHING FOR FOOD

- Am I feeling physical hunger? Do I feel stomach pangs and hollowness? What number am I at on the hunger/fullness scale?
- Am I craving a specific food? If yes, then my hunger must be emotion based. What number am I at on the hunger/fullness scale?

- Can I delay eating this food by engaging myself with another pleasurable activity until my craving dissipates?
- If I eat this portion of food, I realize that my mood will only be uplifted for a few brief seconds. Do the benefits of eating this portion outweigh the negative aspects of eating this portion of food?

REFERENCES

1. Garg, N., Wansink, B., & Inman, J.J. (2007). The influence of incidental affect on consumers' food intake. *Journal of Marketing, 71,* 194–206.
2. Miller, R.S. (1999). Emotion. In V.J. Derlaga, B.A. Winstead, & W.H. Jones (Eds.), *Personality: Contemporary Theory and Research* (pp. 405–431). Chicago: Nelson-Hall.
3. Lazarus, R.S. (1984). On the primacy of cognition. *American Psychologist, 39,* 124–129.
4. Zajonc, R.B. (1980). Feeling and thinking: Preferences need no inferences. *American Psychologist, 35,* 151–175.
5. James, W. (1890). *Principles of Psychology* (Vol. 1). London, UK: Macmillan.
6. Lange, C.J. (1887). *Ueber Gemuthsbewgungen*, Liepzig: T. Thomas.
7. Tooby, J., & Cosmides, L. (1990). On the universality of human nature and the uniqueness of the individual: The role of genetics and adaptation. *Journal of Personality, 58,* 17–67.
8. Allport, G.W. (1937). *Personality: A Psychological Interpretation.* New York: Holt, Rinehart & Winston.
9. Averill, J.R. (1997). The emotions: An integrative account. In R. Hogan, J. Johnson, & S. Briggs (Eds.), *Handbook of Personality Psychology* (pp. 513–541). San Diego: Academic Press.
10. Russell, J.A. (1983). Pancultural aspects of the human conceptual organization of emotions. *Journal of Personality and Social Psychology, 45,* 1281–1288.
11. Larsen, R.J., & Diener, E. (1987). Affect intensity as an individual difference characteristic: A review: *Journal of Research in Personality, 2,* 1–39.
12. Pressman, S.D., & Cohen, S. (2005). Does positive affect influence health? *Psychological Bulletin, 131,* 925–971.
13. Eaton, L.G., & Funder, D.C. (2001). Emotional experience in daily life: Valence, variability and rate of change. *Emotion, 1,* 413–421.
14. Timmerman, G.M., & Acton, G.J. (2001). The relationship between basic needs satisfaction and emotional eating. *Issues in Mental Health Nursing, 22,* 691–701.
15. Van Strien, T., Frijters, J., Bergers, G., & Defares, P. (1986). The Dutch Eating Behaviour Questionnaire (DEBQ) for assessment of restrained, emotional and external eating. *International Journal of Eating Disorders, 5,* 295–315.
16. Heatherton, T.F., & Baumeister, R.F. (1991). Binge eating as an escape from self-awareness. *Psychological Bulletin, 110,* 86–108.
17. Heatherton, T.F., Herman, C.P., & Polivy, J. (1992). Effects of distress on eating: The importance of ego involvement. *Journal of Personality and Social Psychology, 62,* 101–103.

18. Ganley, R.M. (1989). Emotion and eating in obesity: A review of the literature. *International Journal of Eating Disorders, 8*, 343-361.
19. Christensen, L. (1993). Effects of eating behavior on mood: A review of the literature. *International Journal of Eating Disorders, 14*, 171-183.
20. Wansink, B., & SeaBum, P. (2000). Accounting for taste: Prototypes that predict preference. *Journal of Database Marketing, 7*(4), 308-320.
21. Blair, A. J., Lewis, V. J., & Booth, D.A. (1990). Does emotional eating interfere with success in attempts at weight control? *Appetite, 15*(2), 151-157.
22. Ganley, R. M. (1989). Emotion and eating in obesity: A review of the literature. *International Journal of Eating Disorders, 8*, 343-361.
23. Geliebter, A., & Aversa, A. (2003). Emotional eating in overweight, normal weight and underweight individuals. *Eating Behaviors, 3*, 341-347.
24. Ruderman, A.J., (1983). Obesity, anxiety, and food consumption. *Addictive Behaviors, 8*, 235-242.
25. Schachter, S., Goldman, R., & Gordon, A. (1968). Effects of fear, food deprivation and obesity on eating. *Journal of Personality and Social Psychology, 10*, 91-97.
26. Stone, A.A., & Brownell, K.D., 1994. The stress-eating paradox: Multiple daily measurements in adult males and females. *Psychology and Health 13*, 211-219.
27. Meisel, R.L., Hays, T.C., Del Paine, S.N., & Luttrel, Y.R., (1990). Induction of obesity by group housing in female Syrian hamsters. *Physiology & Behavior, 47*, 815-817.
28. Willner, P., Benton, D., Brown, E., Cheeta, S., Davies, G., Morgan, J., et al. (1998). "Depression" increases "craving" for sweet rewards in animal and human models of depression and craving. *Psychopharmacology, 136*, 272-283.
29. Lieberman, H.R., Wurtman, J.J., & Chew, B. (1986). Changes in mood after carbohydrate consumption among obese individuals. *American Journal of Clinical Nutrition, 44*, 772-778.
30. Wurtman, R. J. & Wurtman, J. J. (1989). Carbohydrates and depression. *Scientific American, 260*, 68-75.
31. Johnson, C., & Larson, R. (1982). Bulimia: An analysis of moods and behavior. *Psychosomatic Medicine, 44*, 341-351.
32. Thayer, R.E. (1987). Energy, tiredness, and tension effects of a sugar snack versus moderate exercise. *Journal of Personality and Social Psychology, 52*, 119-125.
33. Hetherington, M.M., & Macdiarmid, J.I. (1993). "Chocolate addiction": A preliminary study of its description and its relationship to problem eating. *Appetite, 2*, 233-246.
34. Macdiarmid, J.I., & Hetherington, M.M. (1995). Mood modulation by food: An explanation of affect and cravings in "chocolate addicts." *British Journal of Clinical Psychology, 34*, 129-138.
35. Hill, A.J., Weaver, C.F., & Blundell, J.E., (1991). Food craving, dietary restraint and mood. *Appetite, 17*, 187-197.
36. Wurtman, R. J. & Wurtman, J. J. (1989). Carbohydrates and depression. *Scientific American, 260*, 68-75.
37. Hill, A.J., Weaver, C.F., & Blundell, J.E. (1991). Food craving, dietary restraint and mood. *Appetite, 17*, 187-197.
38. Christensen, L., Kreitsch, K., White, B., & Stagner, B. (1985). Impact of dietary change on emotional distress. *Journal of Abnormal Psychology, 94*, 565-579.

39. Kreitsch, K., Christensen, L., & White, B. (1988). Prevalence, presenting symptoms, and psychological characteristics of individuals experiencing a diet-related mood-disturbance. *Behavior Therapy, 19,* 593–604.
40. Christensen, L., & Burrows, R. (1990). Dietary treatment of depression. *Behavior Therapist, 21*, 183–193.
41. Wansink, B., & SeaBum, P. (2000). Accounting for taste: Prototypes that predict preference. *Journal of Database Marketing, 7*(4), 308–320.

Section III

EVOLUTIONARY PROCESSES

Chapter 8

Evolutionary Instincts and Eating Patterns

LEARNING OBJECTIVES

By the end of this chapter, the reader will be able to:

1. Understand how evolutionary instincts can affect adherence to an eating plan.
2. Identify instinctual tendencies that lead to over- and undereating behaviors and taste preferences.
3. Apply strategies that will counteract these defunct adaptations, to facilitate adherence to an eating plan.

Is This Safe to Eat?

This is a question that we ask ourselves many times upon going into the refrigerator and pulling out a 2-week-old pound of graying ground sirloin or even a suspicious looking head of lettuce. How do we know when a specific food is safe to consume? Many evolutionary psychologists credit our ancestors for taking care of this dilemma for us, so we do not need to go through a trial-and-error process.

Evolutionary researchers believe that the mechanisms that underlie disgust and food aversions in humans were designed to find certain smells and tastes more aversive than others.

These mechanisms exist because they consistently solved specific problems of survival over evolutionary history. As we know, humans consume a wide variety of plant and animal substances. However, not all such substances are safe to eat. Many plants contain natural toxins, and many animal products are full of parasites that can cause sickness and ultimately death. The psychological mechanisms underlying disgust and food aversions function to reduce the likelihood of ingesting dangerous plant and animal substances.

These mechanisms process the stimuli through sight, touch, taste, and smell of plant and animal substances. Next, the inputs are processed according to a set of decision rules and procedures, such as:

1. Avoid plant substances that taste or smell bitter or especially pungent (indicating high concentrations of plant toxins).[1]
2. Avoid animal substances that emit smells suggestive of spoilage (indicating high levels of toxin-producing bacteria).[2]
3. Avoid foods that one has become sick after consuming in the past.[3]
4. Avoid foods that were not part of one's diet in the first few years of life (especially if it is an animal product).[4]

When relevant decision rules are met, behavioral output is then generated, manifested by specific facial expressions, physical withdrawal from the toxic stimuli, nausea, gagging, spitting, and vomiting.

This output is very adaptive in that it solves the problem of avoiding consumption of harmful substances and of expelling these substances from the body as rapidly as possible if they have been consumed.

EVOLUTIONARY PSYCHOLOGY

One of the newer subdisciplines that has emerged in the last 15 years in the field of psychology is evolutionary psychology. Evolutionary psychology entails the application of the principles and knowledge of evolutionary biology to psychological theory and research. The discipline's basic assumption is that the human brain is composed of numerous specialized mechanisms that were shaped by natural selection over long periods of time to solve the recurrent problems faced by our ancestors.[5] Some of these problems include choosing which foods to eat, developing social hierarchies, dividing investment among offspring, and selecting mates. Evolutionary psychology focuses on understanding these information-processing problems, developing models of the brain-mind tools that may have evolved to solve them, and testing these models in a research setting.[6,7]

EVOLUTIONARY PSYCHOLOGY'S EXPLANATION FOR OBESITY

In the following section you will be introduced to several evolutionary explanations for Western culture's rise in obesity. The explanations are based on holdover evolutionary instincts that were adaptive for our ancestors when food was scarce. Now, in Western society with its abundance of food, these instincts no longer serve a purpose, yet contribute to the counter-productive process of obesity.

Lifestyle

There are many eating behavior patterns that within the framework of evolutionary psychology can be readily explained. For instance, the causal relationship of obesity in the Western culture is explained in the following manner. In our ancestors' time, obtaining sufficient food and nutrition was a daily trial, because life was physically rigorous. Evolutionary psychologists believe that the human body evolved so to become highly efficient at storing excess energy from excess food intake. This excess food could be used at later intervals when food was not available (e.g., during droughts, harsh winter weather). Life has dramatically changed in the Western lifestyle with food that is plentiful and regularly available for consumption. Now with copious amounts of food readily available, it has made physical daily demands very low for people in the Western culture. Due to the striking lifestyle change, obesity is now at an all-time high in Western society. Seventy-two million Americans are considered obese, according to a survey conducted in 2005–2006 by the National Center for Health Statistics and incidences of obesity have increased 61 percent in the period from 1991 to 2000.[8] Interestingly, Australia, another Western society, is one of the most obese countries in the world, as 25% of the children in the country are overweight or obese.[9] Evolutionary psychologists believe, due to these rising statistics, that our dramatic cultural evolution has no longer made the internal storing up of excess food adaptive, thus giving rise to the phenomenon of obesity.[10]

Another lifestyle change that has evolved that affects eating behavior is the context in which a person eats. Originally, humans were solitary eaters and would eat upon finding prey or food such as berries or nuts. As humans evolved and civilizations developed, they no longer ate on the run without companions. Food was brought back to shelters and many times shared with kin. Specific eating areas within shelters were developed with eating rituals included. Think about all of the eating rituals and traditions that exist today that are associated with eating: Eating with utensils, organizing foods on the plate, mixing foods on the plate, peeling fruits or vegetables, eye contact with others at the meal, and conversation are just a few of these rituals. All of these rituals and having multiple companions at the meal distract the eater from their main purpose of eating. Due to these distractions, a person is less sensitive to the cues that the brain and stomach send for satiation and "fullness." When one misses these signals, overeating can occur. Research indicates that the longer the meal, the more people tend to eat at that meal.[11] Additionally, the amount of food people consume at a meal is directly and strongly related to the number of people sharing the meal. Food consumption was found to increase by 28 percent when one other person is present at the meal and increases steadily to 71 percent when the number of companions is six or more.[12] Eating with other people also introduces other powerful social effects. In one study, people were given two bowls of crackers: one containing goldfish crackers and one containing animal crackers. The participants were much more likely to eat the type of crackers that the person they were speaking to was eating, without having any awareness that they were copying the other person. Moreover, people subsequently reported that they preferred the crackers the other person had eaten, without recognizing that their preference was influenced by the other person.[13]

Urban Design

Evolutionary psychologists also attribute Western culture's rising obesity rate to urban design. They state that when cities spread out, so too do its occupants' waistlines. Researchers site cities such as Charleston, West Virginia, or Fort Wayne, Indiana, as their proof.[14] These two U.S. cities have the highest obesity rates and at the same time have less than 3,000 people per square mile occupying the city. More specifically, research has indicated that cities in which people drive to work, to school, and to the food court at the local mall all contribute to obesity in the United States.[15,16] These results are very relevant for urban planners, who have long argued that denser communities are healthier because they facilitate social interaction, because they encourage more daily physical activity. These studies lay the blame in an entirely new framework lifestyle, instead of at the feet of food manufacturers and fast food restaurants that produce and prepare high-calorie foods. Researchers say that two-thirds of the United States is comprised of less-dense urban communities and this adds 6 pounds to the average person.[17] Urban planners should keep in mind that they need to design communities that promote a healthy lifestyle. The implications of sprawling designs on individual health are long ranging; many people in U.S. communities cannot walk even if they wanted to because workplaces are too far apart to permit walking and too spread out to make public transportation practical and economical. Public transportation systems in which residents could walk to and from the bus or subway and leave additional space on the roads for bicycle lanes could be part of an optimal solution. Another solution would be to have mixed zoning statutes that allowed homes, stores, and offices to be in close vicinity so that people could walk to work and do their errands as well.

Ewing and his colleagues examined more than 200,000 Americans living in 448 counties in major metropolitan areas. They calculated the degree of sprawl in each county and then assessed some key health characteristics. The researchers found that people who lived in sprawling neighborhood communities, for the most part, walked less and had less of an opportunity to stay fit.[18]

Food Preferences

In the framework of evolutionary psychology, obesity can also be explained with regard to evolved taste preferences. Consider that there is a strong disposition among many people for sweet-tasting foods. Evolutionary psychologists cite that foods high in sugar, salt, and fat were all in short supply in our ancestral habitats, thus causing our ancestors to develop a predisposition to eat foods with these qualities whenever they were present to maximize their fitness.[19] These researchers believe that we have inherited our ancestors' predispositions to eat these types of foods when they are available. Due to this inherited behavior, we are easy prey for fast food restaurants, which offer foods with all of these qualities on their menus.

Farb and Armelagos in their 1980 book, *Consuming Passions: The Anthropology of Eating*, trace our food preferences back to when humans mainly consumed sea-dwelling creatures.[20] During that time, humans consumed food with great amounts of sea water to facilitate the digestion process and the food's passage in the mouth through the esophagus. The sea water helped to break and soften the food prior to entering the gut or stomach cavity. After humans made the transition from sea to land, much of the food found on land was plants high in starch with tough cellulous and so was difficult to digest without the presence of a catalyst such as water.

To facilitate that part of the digestion process, society developed a wide variety of liquids and foods to serve this purpose. Think about the butter that you habitually put on your dinner roll or bread. This fatty substance not only enhances the taste of one's bread, but serves the purpose of easing its transition down the esophagus. Pancake syrup serves the same purpose, while adding dozens of extra calories to one's meal. Sodas, juices, salad dressings, ketchup, and other condiments are meal supplements that we unconsciously partake of that contribute to Western society's rising obesity rate. Farb discusses our transition from a four-legged mammal to an upright mammal as a factor that ultimately affected our food choices and preferences.[21] As a four-legged mammal, one was limited to the foods that one could find or attack in that prone position (e.g., plants, nuts, berries, other small animals). After transitioning into the upright position, humans had two hands free to carry weapons, help climb, gather foods, and more recently farm. Suddenly, with this change, our diet dramatically changed, because we had more choice over the foods that we consumed. Foods that were rarely attainable suddenly became available. We could choose what foods to gather, store, and consume. Foods that produced a pleasurable taste sensation and could be easily chewed were chosen more often. Many times these types of foods had higher fat and sugar content. Farb points out that learning how to roast foods added to the palatability and fondness for a food.[22] On the other hand, the discovery of cooking, baking, and roasting foods also chemically transformed these foods, many times not in the best nutritional way. Consider wheat, for instance. This food has been milled for thousands of years, but in the 1870s, with the advent of new equipment, millers were able to create a pure white wheat devoid of the most nutritious part, the germ. Due to the lack of the germ, flour now contains less nutrients including vitamin B, folic acid, and potassium. Also, adulterants were added to wheat products to enhance its palatability and consumer appeal. *Adulterants* can be artificial or natural substances that serve to thicken or thin the food, preserve it, or enhance its taste or color. Sugar is the most common leading food additive, with salt being the second most common. Even though salt is the second most common additive, it is more dangerous than sugar because it can lead to high blood pressure, kidney failure, stroke, and heart disease. Studies of existing hunter-gather societies show that these individuals only consume the salt that occurs naturally in their foods.[23] Interestingly, these individuals never develop high blood pressure even in old age. Until our modern era, salt was an extremely rare commodity and was bartered and traded with almost as much enthusiasm as gold. Salt was valued for its ability to preserve fish and meat for long periods of time. Now salt is so abundant in our diets that the average American consumes 5 teaspoons full of it a day, whereas our bodies only require barely 1/4 teaspoon of it.[24] Most of us are familiar with foods that contain salt, but what we don't recognize are items that food manufacturers hide salts in such as cereals, breads, puddings, and almost all canned soups and canned vegetables. This overconsumption of salt in modern diets puts our bodies in a state of mineral imbalance because our bodies did not evolve to tolerate such high levels of sodium.

Prior to the surplus of salt in our world, the human body was accustomed to an abundance of potassium from sources of fresh fruit, now the opposite has occurred. The lack of potassium in our diets directly affects the contractions of our muscles and that of our heart. The imbalance of sodium and potassium causes an accumulation of water to build up, causing an increase in the blood's volume, pressure, and ultimately heart rate. Hence, processed foods, which consist of high levels of salt and low levels of potassium, worsen the situation. These transitions have caused our diet to change from a diet of balance related to scavenging and forging for food to an unbalanced diet of convenient and preferred foods.

In the United States, 70 percent of deaths are linked in some way to poor eating habits and nutrition. These health and eating issues lead to coronary heart disease, adult diabetes, stroke, and high blood pressure.[25] Farb presents the finding that poor nutrition in the United States continues to occur within the last century even though there is an abundance of food. In addition, there has been an increase in this last century in the proportion of calories derived from fat. Most of the carbohydrates consumed in the United States originally came from complex carbohydrates (e.g., whole grains, vegetables and fruit); now these carbohydrates come mostly from refined sugar.

Seasons

Evolutionary psychologists also believe that the seasons of the year contribute to our present-day obesity trend. De Castro's research indicates that people show a seasonal rhythm with regard to their eating patterns.[26] In the fall, there is a marked increase in the populations' total caloric consumption, especially from carbohydrates. According to de Castro, people tend to eat about 200 calories more each day during the fall (excluding the Thanksgiving and Christmas holidays). This calculates to 3–4 extra pounds a year. This pattern is associated with an increase in meal size and a greater rate of eating. De Castro believes that this eating pattern was at one time adaptive for our ancestors because it prepared them for the potential winter famine. During the fall harvest, food is plentiful, thus allowing our ancestors to put on weight to store up for the long winter months. In addition, humans have a tendency to eat whenever food is present. This may be due to our ancestors' feeling of not knowing where their next meal would come from.

Time of Day

The time of day has also been theorized in an evolutionary context to affect our eating habits. Circadian rhythms are our 24-hour biological cycles that govern more than our waking and sleeping. They affect when we are born, when we die, and when we eat. Our body's rhythms are controlled by a "master clock" located in a small region of the brain called the suprachiasmatic nucleus.

This region works like a conductor, striking up one portion of the body's orchestra as another quiets down, taking its main cue from light signals in order to stay synchronized with the hours of the day. The body's hormones surge and ebb in response to this mechanism's commands and our cells even grow faster during certain hours of the day. Circadian rhythms also affect aspects such as birth. Evolution has timed hormones to trigger labor and birth at night, when the mother and her newborn would be less vulnerable to predators. Statistics have supported this idea as natural deliveries occur more frequently in the hours after midnight than during the afternoon. Death also seems to be affected by the time of day, frequently occurring in the morning. This phenomenon occurs because our blood pressure is lowest around 3 AM. When dawn breaks and we get up from bed, our blood pressure rises sharply, increasing the risks of heart attacks and strokes between 8 AM and noon.

Specifically relevant to this textbook, circadian rhythms are believed to signal the onset of eating behavior, especially at night. *Night eating syndrome* is a disorder in which individuals regularly wake one to three times a night to eat, consuming more than half their daily calories during these episodes.[27] Kasof believes that these individuals feel less inhibited in eating when the light is very dim or nonexistent. Kasof conducted two studies with college students, with 245 and 156 students in each respectively; about 20 percent of the students were overweight. Kasof found that those students who were concerned about weight loss were less likely to engage in binge eating if they ate in bright light. Dimmer light, however, increased the risk of binge eating behavior. However, in those without weight concerns, there was no difference in eating behavior. Among 12 students who scored beyond the cutoff for the diagnosis of bulimia, they all preferred dimmer light conditions for eating.

Interestingly, night binge eating does not appear to be a uniquely human tendency. Other species may binge far more often than we do. Predators, uncertain when they will make their next kill, tend to gorge themselves after a successful hunt. Furthermore, early humans—as do many animals—instinctively hunted at twilight or night because their prey was more likely to be caught off guard in a dim setting. Evolutionary psychologists believe that night hunting and bingeing was an adaptive behavior for early humans, thus prompting a circadian rhythm to be developed, signaling a nighttime eating instinct. In present-day Western culture, with copious amounts of food available 24 hours a day, this once-adaptive behavior serves no purpose. Evolutionary psychologists believe, however, that some individuals still display this eating tendency as a holdover from ancestral times.

As additional research is conducted to determine the causes of night eating syndrome, it is believed that it may also be a stress disorder in which the mood declines in the evening and continues to decline throughout the night.[28] Current therapy includes antidepressants that have been shown to help within 2 weeks of beginning the medication. Another theory posits that the person eats to promote sleep because many are afflicted with insomnia. They also tend to consume carbohydrates, possibly to inhibit stress hormones and increase serotonin levels. Stunkard stated, "I think they are eating to medicate themselves because the eating is very high in carbohydrates, and carbohydrates are likely to increase the serotonin in the brain, and that stimulates sleep."[29]

EVOLUTIONARY PSYCHOLOGY'S EXPLANATION FOR ANOREXIA NERVOSA IN WESTERN SOCIETY

A Rationing Instinct

The evolutionary explanation for obesity in Western culture seems very intuitive, so now we will turn toward researchers' account for the opposite problem, anorexia nervosa. Evolutionary psychologists look back to human evolution and realize that it would not have been adaptive always to eat everything available. Instead, it would have been wise to ration during times when food was scarce, while eating heavily during times when food was more plentiful.[30] These psychologists believe that the ability to go without food would have been very adaptive for one's survival. This would have been a difficult quality to develop, however, because it would be in direct opposition of our natural instinct to gratify hunger instead of delay it. Further, evolutionary psychologists believe that this behavior of going without food for the benefit of the entire group was reinforced by the group members, because humans evolved in social groups. Within the context of the evolutionary perspective, eating behavior evolved to meet the individual and social needs of humans. In other words, the eating behavior of our ancestors was a complex interplay of pleasure and gratification that was tempered by higher reasoning and social norms that emphasized eating a minimum for current survival in order to help maximize the long-term likelihood of survival. Guisinger also adds that this phenomenon is seen in the animal kingdom because many animals are able to "turn off" eating if they have something more important to do. For instance, gray whales are able to turn off their eating instincts while migrating, even though food is plentiful.

Individual Differences

In today's society, evolutionary psychologists posit that individual differences in personality characteristics contribute to whether an individual will manifest this evolved "eat the minimum" eating behavior. These psychologists suggest that if an individual has an overactive superego (e.g., conscience) or oversusceptibility to social messages about eating less, then they are predisposed to engaging in anorexic or bulimic behavior patterns.[31]

Reproductive Status

Singh offers another evolutionary-based explanation for anorexia nervosa, proposing that the gynoid (lower body) fat distribution or the waist-to-hip ratio (WHR) of females is a critical and universal cue in signaling reproductive value to males.[32] According to Singh, a typical and healthy range for WHR in females is from 0.67 to 0.80.[33] This reasoning stems from evidence indicating links between the WHR and mechanisms affecting female health and reproductive status (such as puberty, ovarian disease, menstrual irregularity, diabetes, and mortality). A WHR in the ideal range should thus be conceptualized as being most attractive to males because it signals high-reproductive capability and accurately signals health in terms of absence of disease.[34] Singh believes that males have evolved mechanisms to detect the WHR of females to evaluate their health and reproductive capacity. The processes of mate attraction and mate selection have been significantly advanced by the introduction of the concept of "mate value."[35] This idea is based on the assumption that individual members of a given species are not equally valuable to members of the opposite sex as mates. Consistent with this view, the female mate value is highly related with her reproductive potential and thus males will be sensitive to visual evidence of youth and good health, both of which are highly relevant to female fertility.[36] The human female develops a distinctive fat distribution following puberty that results in the hourglass or so called "wasp-waist" shape, typical of nubile women. To propagate, our male ancestors had to be visually perceptive to these physical cues of fertility. Interestingly, it has been hypothesized that to avoid rearing another man's offspring, men developed an aversion to even a slight thickening of the waist.[37] This aversion would most likely be directed toward novel females and should be particularly relevant to the male's choice of a long-term mate. Participants in experiments using line drawings of female figures in which the ratio of the hips to the waist was subtly altered, showed a strong preference for females with the thinnest waist. The most attractive female WHR was judged to be 0.7 to 0.8 both by males and females.[38]

Further, the present hypothesis suggests that what we now call eating disorders are a manifestation of "runaway" female intrasexual competition (a self-destructive competition between females to secure a mate by maintaining a youthful/nubile physique). This process is a phenomenon that entails phenotypic change as a result of environmental factors. Reproductive potential (RP) in females is mainly a function of age and decreases with advancing years down to zero at menopause. A female's maximum RP occurs 3 to 4 years following puberty; this matches the time the nubile female body takes its full shape. Hence, the newly nubile female will have a higher RP than at any other time during her lifetime. It would make sense that males would be particularly attracted to females who display the nubile shape. It has indeed been suggested that across cultures, the female shape found to be most sexually attractive is that of the nubile female.[39] It is also argued that, in the ancestral environment, the female's shape provided a generally accurate indicator of her reproductive history. Thus, the visual cue representing this relatively slender nubile shape became a significant and highly effective part of the human female's strategy for physical attractiveness. Males developed a "taste" for the visual cue of the nubile female in the ancestral environment and sought out these women. It was believed these women would have had a reproductive edge through the acquisition of "breeding rights" for the longest possible period of a certain female's reproductive life.

Therefore, it is theorized that an adaptation involving a behavioral strategy that focuses on the preservation or the restoration of the nubile shape (the drive toward thinness) would have given females who possessed it a reproductive edge in the ancestral environment. This drive for nubility is a form of female intrasexual competition designed by selection to secure the best possible long-term mate through the signaling of high RP. Eating disorders may be described as a state of runaway female intrasexual competition in which the originally adaptive strategy spirals out of control becoming self-destructive.

Also, the human characteristics of language and cognitive processing have greatly enhanced the process of social comparison, thus facilitating the destructive potential of this runaway/out of control feedback loop. The idea that eating disorders are the by-product of intrasexual competition between females would be consistent with the clinical observation that the symptoms of the disorder can be highly reactive to the social context and may show complete remission by changing one's sociocultural setting.[40] The last evolutionary-based theory of anorexia nervosa is the one posited by Voland and Voland.[41] This theory, as does Singh's WHR theory, links the eating disorder to a female's state of fertility, but in a different manner. The researchers suggest that anorexia nervosa is an emergency strategy that has evolved through selection that comes into play to suppress reproduction when other controls fail. This is achieved through the reduction of the critical fat mass to below the threshold for ovulation. Situations such as drought, war, and famine are considered to be logical states of emergency in which a woman might engage in this type of behavior. The researchers suggest that certain features within present day environment have led to the increase in the use of this emergency strategy.

It is important to note here that anorexia nervosa is a multicausal psychological disorder. The evolutionary psychologist's theory of development is only one of many possible causative theories.

STRATEGIES TO COUNTERACT INSTINCTUAL EATING PATTERNS

Several evolutionary-based theories have been discussed related to over- and undereating. At this point in the chapter, psychological strategies will be given to counteract these once-adaptive, but now-defunct eating behaviors. Half of the battle is recognizing the origins of maladaptive eating behaviors and the purpose that these behaviors once served.

Activity Level

It is important to be cognizant of the fact that our ancestors led a very physically rigorous lifestyle, hunting their food between each meal and growing their own foods. Our Western lifestyle is dramatically sedentary in comparison to our ancestors and even in comparison to that of our relatives who lived 60–70 years ago. We tend to conceptualize exercise as a recent fad or trend, but the truth of the matter is that our ancestors exercised way beyond the level of the average person in Western society. Exercise was a necessity for our ancestors to survive as they literally earned each meal. By earning each meal, our ancestors were able to keep their eating behavior in equal proportion to their exercise behavior, resulting in a state of harmony. By making it a point each day to keep your ratio of exercise behavior to eating behavior equivalent, then states of overeating or undereating will not occur and a healthier body weight will be easier to attain and maintain.

One way we can do this is to track our activity just as we would our food intake. A study conducted by researchers at the University of Pittsburgh found that 275 minutes of moderate physical activity per week was sufficient to maintain significant weight loss (10 percent of initial body weight) even 2 years poststudy.[42] Another recommendation to encourage an equal balance of activity to eating is to purchase and wear a pedometer. Track how many steps you take on average over a 1-week time frame. Take that number and multiply it by 1.2. This would then be the goal number of steps that you would want to work on achieving over that same time frame. Studies have shown that to maintain a healthy body weight, 10,000 steps per day should be your goal. To lose weight, 12,000–15,000 steps per day is recommended. Tracking activity and food intake is the best way to determine if your energy equation is balanced. When it is, your body will be in the state of balance and harmony that it was originally designed to be in.

Urban Design

Now that a link has been shown between sprawling neighborhoods and obesity, one might want to consider the layout of your own neighborhood. Are you living in an extremely dense environment so that you are forced to walk or bike everywhere? Or are you living in a less-dense environment in which you drive to all of your daily destinations? Chances are if you are living in a densely packed city, you are getting your daily exercise and your ratio of food to exercise is in a state of balance. However, if you reside in a sprawling neighborhood, it is likely that your food-to-exercise ratio is skewed in the direction of food consumption. Mapping out some destinations within your residential neighborhood where you can walk (wearing your pedometer) or bike to (track the number of minutes toward accumulating 275 minutes/week) on a regular basis would be advisable or compensating for that lack of exercise through a daily workout routine would be optimal. Attend city planning meetings to see where walking and biking trails or lanes could be constructed. Start a "walking school bus" in your neighborhood where a few adults walk a specific route to school and "pick up" children on their way.

Eating Rituals

As previously mentioned, the rituals in today's eating environment have also been linked to obesity. Today's eating environment is no longer solitary, but full of distractions from the task at hand: eating. From an evolutionary standpoint, one would want to minimize all potential distractions at the eating table, so to not miss those "all-full" signals that the brain and stomach emit. Of course, eliminating family members and friends from the eating table is not advisable, but ensure that the conversation stays "light" and does not become emotionally charged. Turn off the television and dine at the table. Serve your dining companions' meals directly from the stove and not family style from the table. When plates of food are left on the table, it is easy to mindlessly serve second and third portions. With the extra food remaining on the stove, one is less likely to get up during the meal (at least without a great deal of conscious thought) to retrieve seconds or thirds. Practice eating slowly and putting your eating utensils down in between bites. Research studies have found that those who eat quickly consume many more total calories than those who eat more slowly.[43] Also ensure that the lighting at the dining table is bright so everyone can be acutely aware of the portions that they are consuming. This technique will also help those individuals who are prone to night eating syndrome.

Condiment Usage

As mentioned earlier, condiments such as butter and salad dressing served as catalysts to help in the early stages of the digestion process for foods that were tough to swallow and digest such as breads and fibrous foods. With this now known, write down all of your daily condiment usage. You will probably find that it is quite high, and that these condiments are also high in sugar, calories, or salt. Next, write down healthier alternatives that you could use in place of these condiments to help in the swallowing and digestion process. Water is an ideal alternative and will be discussed extensively in an upcoming chapter.

Another alternative would be to cut foods that are difficult to swallow into smaller pieces, rather than relying on condiments to ease their transitions down the esophagus. Also, taking time to chew each bite of food thoroughly before swallowing will help to eliminate the use of sugary or salty condiments.

UNDERSTANDING ONE'S INSTINCTS

Whether it be the time of day, the seasons, or an unnatural instinct to refrain from eating, understanding the origins of these defunct instincts is the key to combating them and adhering to a balanced nutritional eating plan. Taking control of your environment and not letting your environment control you is of the utmost importance.

You Diagnose It

ADHERENCE SCENARIO 1

Terry calls herself a "carpool mom" because she feels like she is constantly in her car, driving her children to school, music lessons, social events, and sports practices. Terry has gained significant weight since she became a carpool mom even though she insists that she eats the same amount and types of foods that she did prior to becoming a chauffeur mom.

1. Give an evolutionary-based explanation for Terry's recent weight gain.
2. Develop a long-range plan (that is consistent with your answer to Question 1) to address both Terry's weight gain and carpooling dilemmas.

ADHERENCE SCENARIO 2

Kenny has a tendency to wake up two to three times each night and consume over 2,000 calories. He also notes that when he and his girlfriend dine at their favorite dimly lit Italian restaurant that he always orders and consumes more than all of his other meals combined during the day.

1. Give an evolutionary-based explanation for Kenny's bingeing behavior.

2. Develop a long-range plan (that is consistent with your answer to Question 1) to address Kenny's bingeing behavior.

Review

- ✓ Evolutionary psychology entails the application of the principles and knowledge of evolutionary biology to psychological theory and research.

- ✓ Evolutionary psychologists believe that the human body evolved to become highly efficient at storing excess energy from excess food intake. This excess food could be used at later intervals when food was not available (e.g., during droughts, harsh winter weather).

- ✓ Originally, humans were solitary eaters. Today, people have developed many eating rituals involving other companions during the meal. The amount of food one consumes at a meal is directly and strongly related to the number of people sharing the meal.

- ✓ Evolutionary psychologists also attribute Western culture's rising obesity rate to its urban design. More specifically, research indicates that cities in which people drive to work, to school, and to the food court at the local mall, all contribute to obesity in the United States.

- ✓ Obesity can also be explained, in the framework of evolutionary psychology, with regard to evolved taste preferences. Consider the fact that there is a strong disposition among many people for sweet-tasting foods. Evolutionary psychologists cite that foods high in sugar, salt, and fat were all in short supply in our ancestral habitats, thus causing our ancestors to develop a predisposition to eat foods with these qualities whenever they were present to maximize their fitness.

- ✓ Research has indicated that people show a seasonal rhythm with regard to their eating patterns. In the fall, there is a marked increase in the populations' total caloric consumption, especially from carbohydrates.

- ✓ The eating behavior of our ancestors was a complex interplay of pleasure and gratification that was tempered by higher reasoning and social norms that emphasized eating a minimum for current survival in order to help maximize the long-term likelihood of survival.

✓ The drive for nubility is a form of female intrasexual competition designed by selection to secure the best possible long-term mate through the signaling of high RP. Eating disorders may be described as a state of runaway female intrasexual competition in which the originally adaptive strategy spirals out of control becoming self-destructive.

D.I.E.T. (Do I Eat This?)

TIPS TO CONSIDER WHEN REACHING FOR A PIECE OF FOOD

- Is my ratio of eating to exercise in proportion today?
- Are the condiments on this food necessary?
- Have I minimized all possible distractions in my eating environment?
- Do I have a tendency to eat this food during a certain time of the day? A certain season?

REFERENCES

1. Profet, M. (1992). Pregnancy sickness as adaptation: A deterrent to maternal ingestion of teratogens. In J.H. Barkow, L. Cosmides, & J. Tooby (Eds.), *The Adapted Mind: Evolutionary Psychology and the Generation of Culture* (pp. 327–365). New York: Oxford University Press.
2. Ibid.
3. Seligman, M., & Hagar, J. (1972). *Biological Boundaries of Learning.* New York: Appleton-Century-Crofts.
4. Cashdan, E. (1994). A sensitive period for learning about food. *Human Nature, 5,* 279–291.
5. Symons, D. (1995). Beauty is in the adaptations of the beholder: The evolutionary psychology of human female sexual attractiveness. In P.R. Abramson & S.D. Pinkerton (Eds.), *Sexual Nature, Sexual Culture* (pp. 80–118). Chicago: University of Chicago Press.
6. Buss, D.M. (1995). Evolutionary psychology: A new paradigm for psychological science. *Psychological Inquiry, 6,* 1–49.
7. Tooby, J., & Cosmides, L. (1992). The psychological foundation of culture. In J.H. Barkow, L. Cosmides, & J. Tooby (Eds.), *The Adapted Mind: Evolutionary Psychology and the Generation of Culture* (pp. 19–137). New York: Oxford University Press.
8. Ogden, C.L., Carroll, M.D., Curtin, L.R., McDowell, M.A., Tabak, C.J., & Flegal, K.M. (2006). Prevalence of overweight and obesity in the United States, 1999–2004. *Journal of the American Medical Association, 295,* 1549–1555.
9. Australasian Society for the Study of Obesity. (2007). Fast Facts-Statistics. Available at: http://www.asso.org.au/home/obesityinfo/stats/fastfacts. Accessed December, 2009.
10. Feist, J., & Feist, G.J. (2002). *Theories of Personality* (5th ed.). New York: McGraw-Hill.

11. Feunekes, G.I., de Graaf, C., & van Staveren, W.A. (1995). Social facilitation of food intake is mediated by meal duration. *Physiology & Behavior, 58,* 551-558.

12. de Castro, J.M., & Brewer, E. (1992). The amount eaten in meals by humans is a power function of the number of people present. *Physiology & Behavior, 51,* 121-125.

13. Chartrand, T.L. (2005). The role of conscious awareness in consumer behavior. *Journal of Consumer Psychology, 15,* 203-210.

14. Ewing, R., Schmid, T., Killingsworth, R., Zlot, A., & Raudenbush, S. (2003). Relationship between urban sprawl and physical activity, obesity, and morbidity. *American Journal of Health Promotion, 18*(1), 47-57.

15. Ibid.

16. Frank, L.D., & Engelke, P. (2005). Multiple impacts of the built environment on public health: Walkable places and the exposure to air pollution. *International Regional Science Review, 28*(2), 193-216.

17. Ibid.

18. Ewing, R., Schmid, T., Killingsworth, R., Zlot, A., & Raudenbush, S. (2003). Relationship between urban sprawl and physical activity, obesity, and morbidity. *American Journal of Health Promotion, 18*(1), 47-57.

19. Farb, P., & Armelagos, G. (2000a). The patterns of eating. In J. Siler, K. Gadbow, & M. Medelevz (Eds.), *The Quill Reader* (pp. 369-372). Fort Worth, TX: Harcourt.

20. Farb, P., & Armelagos, G. (1980). *Consuming Passions: The Anthropology of Eating* Boston, MA: Houghton Mifflin Company.

21. Ibid.

22. Ibid.

23. Ibid.

24. Ibid.

25. Ibid.

26. de Castro, J.M. (1991). Social facilitation of the spontaneous meal size of humans occurs on both weekdays and weekends. *Physiology Behavior, 49,* 1289-1291.

27. Kasof, J. (2002). Indoor lighting preferences and bulimic behavior: An individual differences approach. *Personality and Individual Differences, 32*(3), 383-400.

28. O'Reardon, J.P., Peshek, A., & Allison, K.C. (2005). Night eating syndrome: Diagnosis, epidemiology and management. *CNS Drugs, 12,* 997-1008.

29. Stunkard, A.J. (2006). Disorders of overeating, binge eating disorder and night eating syndrome. *International Journal of Psychopharmacology, 9,* S17-S17.

30. Guisinger, S. (2003). Adapted to famine: Adding an evolutionary perspective on anorexia nervosa. *Psychological Review, 110,* 475-761.

31. Cosmides, L., & Tooby, J. (1997). Dissecting the computational architecture of social inference mechanisms. In: *Characterizing Human Psychological Adaptations* (Ciba Symposium Volume 208). Chichester, UK: Wiley.

32. Singh, D. (1993a). Adaptive significance of female physical attractiveness: Role of waist-to-hips ratio. *Journal of Personality and Social Psychology, 65,* 293-307.

33. Singh, D. (1993b). Body shape and women's attractiveness: The critical role of waist-to hips ratio. *Human Nature, 4,* 297-321.

34. Singh, D. (1995). Female judgment of male attractiveness and desirability for relationships: Role of waist-to-hip ratio and financial status. *Journal of Personality and Social Psychology, 69,* 1089-1101.

35. Symons, D. (1987) An evolutionary approach: Can Darwin's view of life shed light on human sexuality? In J.H. Geer & W.T. O'Donohue (Eds.), *Theories of Human Sexuality* (pp. 91-125). New York: Plenum Press.

36. Buss, D.M. (1987). Sex differences in human mate selection criteria: An evolutionary perspective. In C. Crawford, M. Smith, & D. Krebs (Eds.), *Sociobiology and Psychology: Ideas, Issues and Applications* (pp. 335-351). Mahwah, NJ: Lawrence Erlbaum.

37. Ridley, M. (1993). *The Red Queen: Sex and the Evolution of Human Nature*. London, UK: Viking.

38. Singh, D. (1994). Ideal body shape: Role of body weight and waist-to-hip ratio. *International Journal of Eating Disorders, 16*(3), 283-288.

39. Brown, P.J., & Konner, M. (1987). An anthropological perspective on obesity. *Annals of the New York Academy of Sciences, 499,* 29-46.

40. Raphael, F.J., & Lacey, J.H. (1992). Sociocultural factors in eating disorders. *Annals of Medicine, 24,* 293-296.

41. Voland, E., & Voland, R. (1989). Evolutionary biology and psychiatry: The case for anorexia nervosa. *Ethology and Sociobiology, 10,* 223-240.

42. Jakicic, J.M., Marcus, B.H., Lang, W., & Janney, C. (2002). 24-month effects of exercise weight loss in overweight women. *Archives of Internal Medicine, 168,* 1550-1559.

43. Andrade, A., Minaker, T., & Melanson, K.J. (2004). Eating rate and satiation in lean women. *International Journal of Obesity, 112*(s), A57.

Section IV

PSYCHODYNAMIC PERSPECTIVE

Chapter 9

Psychoanalytic Approach and Eating Patterns

LEARNING OBJECTIVES

By the end of this chapter, the reader will be able to:

1. Understand the basic tenets of Freud's theories.

2. Identify each of the eight defense mechanisms that individuals use to cope with anxiety.

3. Be cognizant about the relationship between childhood development and later adult eating behavior and personality characteristics.

4. Replace existing anxiety-related coping strategies with effective techniques to adhere to a prescribed eating plan.

Talk It Out, Write It Out, Draw It Out

Children do it all the time; adults rarely do: drawing!

Can something so simple as drawing a picture ease one's anxieties? Freud would probably answer "Yes!"

Before Sigmund Freud's ideas came to the forefront of society, it was the societal norm for individuals to keep their worries, anxieties and impulses bottled up inside themselves. Don't ask, don't tell, may well have been the creed. As one can imagine, this was a recipe for disaster and was a time bomb just waiting to explode.

Freud came along and revolutionized that maladaptive norm with his "talking cure." Freud instructed his patients to say whatever came to mind, using words to verbalize all that resided in one's preconscious mind. This was the beginning of the psychoanalytic method. With his eating disorder patients, Freud also had them write freely about whatever was on their mind so to allow them another vehicle to reveal and release their tensions. Freud found this technique especially helpful with these patients because he believed that they used their bodies (eating) rather than their words to express their emotions.

Researchers like Sharon Farber built on Freud's talking and writing therapies and is embarking on additional creative methods, such as drawing, to reach those patients, who are especially resistant to free association.

FOUR KEY COMPONENTS TO PSYCHOANALYTIC THEORY

This chapter is devoted to understanding how the hidden and unconscious portions of one's mind can affect daily behavior, and more specifically, eating behavior. We will be discussing psychoanalysis, which is a group of theories developed by Austrian physician Sigmund Freud (1856–1939) and further developed by other researchers. There are four key ideas that comprise the psychoanalytic theory: psychic determinism, internal structure, psychic conflict, and mental energy.[1] Let's first look at the foundation of Freud's theory, psychic determinism. *Psychic determinism* is the assumption that everything a person thinks or does has a specific cause and this cause most of the time can be found in the mental processes that are hidden in one's unconscious. Research has indicated that only a small part of the mind is available to conscious awareness.[2,3,4] Freud proposed the metaphor that our mind is like an iceberg where only the upper 10 percent of it is visible (i.e., conscious); the remaining 90 percent is submerged under the water and unseen (preconscious and unconscious).[5] We can use the metaphor of an iceberg to help us in understanding Freud's topographical theory (see **Figure 9–1**) According to Freud, there are three levels of consciousness:

1. *conscious*: This is the portion of the mind that holds what you're aware of. You can put into words your conscious experience and you can think about it in a logical manner.

2. *preconscious*: This is one's regular memory. Although things stored here aren't in the conscious, they can be readily brought into conscious.

3. *unconscious*: Freud believed that this portion of the mind was not accessible to awareness. He theorized that one's unconscious was where impulses, feelings, and ideas that are related to anxiety, conflict, and pain were stored. These feelings and impulses, even though they are in storage, exert influence on our behaviors and our conscious awareness.

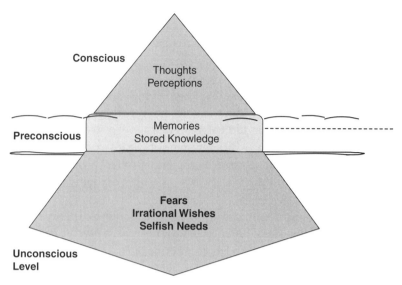

Figure 9–1 Freud's Iceberg Metaphor for the Psyche or Mind.

Freud posited that thoughts pass easily back and forth between the conscious and the preconscious. Also, he believed that thoughts from these two areas can be deposited into the unconscious as well. The thoughts residing in the unconscious can only be known or available through the help of a psychoanalyst, Freud believed.

The second most prominent idea in Freud's theory is internal structure. Freud posited that our mind has an internal structure made of several parts that function independently and sometimes come into conflict with each other. It is important to note that there is a prominent difference between the terms "mind" and "brain." The brain is a physical organ and the mind is the psychological result of what the brain and the body do. According to the psychoanalytic theory, the mind is divided into three parts: the id, ego, and superego. The *id* portion of the mind usually is focused on obtaining instant gratification and is fueled by impulses. The *superego* functions as the moral compass in one's mind, while the *ego* is the rational moderator between the id and the superego. Interestingly, modern psychological research has not found that the mind is actually divided neatly into three distinct parts, however, research does support the concept that the mind consists of separate and independent structures that process different thoughts and motivations at the same time.[6,7]

The Mind's Internal Conflict

The third aspect of the psychoanalytic theory revolves around the concept of psychic conflict or the tension between the id and the superego that the ego is moderating. For instance, suppose your id impulsively wants to indulge in a slice of chocolate cake. Your superego, on the other hand, does not think you should eat it because you need to control your type 2 diabetes. The brunt of the conflict would then fall to your ego to formulate a compromise, such as indulging in a different type of sugar-free dessert. According to Freud, all behavior is motivated by the desire to feel pleasure. That motivation is organized and directed by two instincts: sexuality (*eros*) and aggression (*thanatos*).

The last key assumption that comprises psychoanalytic theory is the apparatus that fuels the mind. Freud refers to this fuel as psychic energy or libido. Freud believed that only a finite amount of this energy is available at any given moment and is only responsible for powering one part of the mind at a time. Psychic energy, in the modern psychoanalytic theory, is considered in terms of mental or computer capacity. One of the aim's of psychoanalysis is to free up more psychic energy, or capacity, for the challenges of daily living by alleviating each one of the client's neurotic conflicts. Freud also posits that not only do humans have a life drive, the libido, but also have a drive toward death and destruction, that is termed thanatos, which results in aggression. Additionally, one's psychological development is the saga of how your life energy or libido is focused in different areas over the course of five developmental stages in life.

Freud's Stage Theory

Freud developed dynamic and psychosocial explanations for human behavior; he also conceptualized the psychosexual stages of development. Freud believed that there are prominent stages in which an individual has a specific need, and if his or her needs are left unmet or overstimulated, according to Freud, there are lasting effects on an individual's behavior. Freud believed that the negative outcomes of each of these stages accounted for an individual's deviance or abnormal behavior. The five psychosexual stages are the oral stage, the anal stage, the phallic stage, the latency stage, and the genital stage.

The first stage that individuals enter is the oral stage. This stage occurs during the first 2 years of life. The mouth is the prominent erogenous zone. Freud believed that an *erogenous zone* was a particular portion of the body from which we seek and gain pleasure. According to Freud, an infant's biggest source of gratification is sucking. As we know, it is very natural to see an infant between the ages of 1 to 2 years constantly putting objects in his or her mouth. The anal stage is next; individuals typically enter it from age 2 to 3. The membranes of the anal area provide the prominent source of pleasurable stimulation because toilet-training is an important developmental stage in this time period of a child's life. Next, the phallic stage occurs from ages 3 to 6. This stage focuses on self-manipulation of the genitals as providing the prominent source of pleasurable stimulation. One typically next encounters the latency stage from age 6 to 12. In this stage, sexual motivations become less important as the child is focused more on developing other skills and engaging in other activities. The last stage of development is the genital stage. This final stage occurs after puberty and continues into adulthood. Optimally, during this stage, the strongest feelings of pleasure come from sexual relationships with other adults.

Freud posited that fulfillment during each stage is important to prevent a person from becoming fixated in any of the stages. *Fixation*, according to Freud, is attaching oneself in an exaggerated or unnatural manner to another individual or thing during that stage of development. Freud stated that a fixation at one specific stage can cause problems in an individual's adult life. Probably the two stages most relevant to eating behavior are the oral and anal stages. For instance, if a person is stuck in the oral stage of development or orally fixated, that person may bite their nails or chew on pencils. Additionally, if an infant is not given adequate oral gratification, he or she may be prone to excessive eating or drinking in their adult life. In the anal stage, if a person had a rigid anal stage by having a tough time being toilet training, Freud believed that this person was more likely to be obsessively neat and obsessive about other aspect such as eating in their adult lives.

DEFENSE MECHANISMS AND ANXIETY

Another facet to Freud's psychoanalytic paradigm is the coping mechanisms that individuals engage in on a daily basis. Freud believed that an important role of the ego is to keep disturbing parts of one's life or mental life away from conscious thought and locked in the unconscious portion of the mind. The ego uses what Freud calls defense mechanisms to keep forbidden impulses and disturbing thoughts suppressed in the unconscious mind. Defense mechanisms are not always foolproof at keeping disturbing thoughts or impulses suppressed, because sometimes words, thoughts, and even actions seep to the surface of our conscious thought. These "behavioral slips" can come forth in a variety of ways such as through humor, accidents or unintentional wordage.

Coping Mechanisms

Coping mechanisms are the way that we deal with minor to major stress and trauma. Some of these processes are unconscious ones, others are learned behavior, and still others are skills we consciously master in order to reduce stress or other strong emotions like depression. Freud believed that not all coping mechanisms are beneficial, and some can actually be very harmful.

Keep in mind that the human body has an interior set of coping mechanisms when it encounters stress. This includes the fight-or-flight reaction to high stress or trauma. A person who perceives stress has an automatic increase in adrenaline, inducing either action or inaction. Other automatic coping strategies can include the way our minds deal with a big onslaught of stress. Some researchers suggest that mental illness is a form of coping mechanism that evolved from certain stressors. For example, multiple personality disorder may result in children who are severely abused. Panic attacks may be the body's coping mechanisms for inappropriate fight-or-flight reactions to minor stressors.

We also develop or learn coping mechanisms as we go through life. Some people gravitate toward coping mechanisms that are helpful, while others choose defense mechanisms that add to one's stress level. For example, individuals who turn to drugs, alcohol, or develop an eating disorder are using unhealthy and dangerous coping methods. A stressed individual who uses exercise to release their stress is utilizing a healthy coping mechanism. We may not always be able to control the amount of adrenaline that pumps through our bodies in stressful situations, but many therapists believe we can learn to control our reaction to it.

Denial and Repression

Here are the defense mechanisms that Freud proposed. The simplest of all defense mechanisms is *denial* in which the ego refuses to acknowledge the source of one's anxiety. This tactic can be an effective short-term tactic, but in the long run, it can be serious due to losing contact with reality.[8] An individual who is 100 pounds overweight, yet refuses to admit that he has a weight problem is using "denial" to keep this uncomfortable fact out of his awareness. A more complex defense mechanism is *repression*. Repression is longer lasting than denial and involves the ego banishing the past from present awareness completely. For example, when Tanisha is confronted by her friends about her ice cream bingeing episode last night, she truthfully answers that she has no recollection of it. Tanisha has pushed her anxiety-provoking episode from her preconscious mind to her unconscious mind where she is unable to access it.

Reaction Formation

An even more complex defense mechanism than repression is a reaction formation. A *reaction formation* keeps forbidden thoughts, feelings, and behaviors out of awareness by initiating their opposites. This process helps to maintain an individual's self-esteem.[9] For instance, if an individual feels that he engages in an unacceptable eating behavior, he may strive to engage in just the opposite behavior in front of others. More specifically, if Marisa feels bad that she overeats at meals, she may eat small portions when dining out with friends.

Projection and Rationalization

To further protect against unwanted impulses, some individuals use the defense mechanism coined as projection. *Projection* involves attributing one's forbidden impulse, thought, or behavior to another individual. The statement "It is not me who eats unhealthy, it is you" exemplifies the projection process. Probably the most commonly used defense mechanism is *rationalization*. In this process, the ego concocts a logically rational reason to defend why the person engaged in the shameful behavior: "I had to eat Patty's homemade cheesecake, because if I did not, she would never forgive me." This rationalization would help to alleviate the shameful feelings one might have for not adhering to a controlled carbohydrate eating plan as part of their diabetes management. The process of trivializing the shameful action can also be part of the rationalization process. "It was just a tiny sliver of cheesecake with hardly any carbohydrates. I'm sure it did not affect my blood sugar level" would be an example of trivializing the shameful behavior.

Intellectualization

An alternative way to deal with an uncomfortable and potentially threatening emotion is by using the defense mechanism of intellectualization. *Intellectualization* can turn an emotional source of anxiety into a distant analytical, intellectual concept, or description. For instance, a surgeon may simply say that the patient "expired" rather than "died" to help distance herself from emotional pain or anxiety—or Dale may say that he "ingested an insignificant amount of gluten" rather than admit that he did not adhere to his eating plan and ate two slices of fresh-baked French bread. By referring to his behavior in this manner, Dale will be able to continue on with his day, feeling a minimal amount of anxiety about not adhering to his gluten-free diet.

Displacement

Another defense mechanism, though less intellectual, is *displacement*. This process involves replacing one object of emotion with another. For instance, the ego will relocate the id's forbidden impulse on another person or object. If one has the desire to binge on sweets, then the ego might redirect this impulse into another activity such as yelling at the TV set. In other words, the impulse is transferred to a safer, more acceptable, outlet.

Sublimation

The last defense mechanism discussed is sublimation. Individuals who use this technique transform their forbidden impulses into constructive behaviors. One's choice of occupation is a natural area to look for one's sublimation tendencies. Some individuals might express their frustrations and forbidden passions by choosing a career as an artist, while an individual who loves to belittle others for not being good enough might choose an occupation as a food or movie critic. It is even possible that an individual who is obsessive about food may become a chef. Freud actually believed that the process of sublimation is a positive process and unlike the other defense mechanisms, sublimation does not really have a downside to it.

Behavioral Slips

As mentioned earlier, defense mechanisms do not consistently keep forbidden impulses suppressed out of awareness, because sometimes they "leak" into our conscious thoughts or behaviors in the form of behavioral slips also known as parapraxes or Freudian slips. Behavioral *slips* are unintentional actions that are caused by the leakage of suppressed impulses. Addressing your current girlfriend by the name of your past girlfriend would be an example of a Freudian slip. Breaking a casserole dish that was left at your house by your boss—who did not give you a good 6-month review—would be another example of a behavioral slip. Freud believed that there are really no accidents; that all behaviors have a deep-rooted cause. Additionally, failure at work, in academics or sports, or to an eating adherence plan can also be a form of a behavioral slip. After failure, you need to ask yourself: Did you really want to succeed or were you, at some unconscious level, wanting to fail for a particular reason? Freud would say that your failure indicates an internal conflict that you might have about winning or being successful that might produce guilt or shame. For example, some individuals who are following an eating plan with the goal of losing excess body fat find ways to self-sabotage their efforts. They may unconsciously prevent themselves from achieving success because their excess weight is "speaking for them." For some individuals, remaining overweight gives them a reason to blame for their failures: "If I wasn't overweight, I would have gotten the promotion" or "If I wasn't overweight, I would be making a higher salary." If they adhered to their eating plan and lost weight, they would no longer have their excess body weight as an excuse for their failures and would then feel inadequate, guilty, or shameful. To avoid experiencing these feelings, they have difficulty adhering to their eating plan and remain overweight.

Humor is a methodical way that we express our forbidden impulses, whereas behavioral slips are uncontrolled. Freud believed that humor or wit was a form of sublimation. If you think about it, much of the humor that we hear around the water cooler or on television is about forbidden topics such as sex and violence. Jokes are an acceptable way to discuss a forbidden impulse in a safe manner. Again, humor from a Freudian vantage point is seen as positive because it allows the uncomfortable impulse to be released and shared in a safe environment.

A CRITIQUE OF THE PSYCHOANALYTIC THEORY

Freud's theories have enjoyed a resurgence in the last few years. For instance, the cover of the March 27, 2006 issue of *Newsweek* had a picture of Freud with the caption: "Freud Is Not Dead. . . . The Couch is Out, but the Culture of Therapy is Everywhere . . . and Science is Taking a New Look at His Theories."[10] Freud's theories have permeated popular culture and many of the terms that we use on a daily basis to categorize ourselves and others ("You are so anal." "You are just in denial about it.") were developed by Freud. Freudian psychoanalysis is seen as one of the first systematic, psychodynamic approaches to show how human psychological processes can result in mental disorders. Freud theorized that some abnormal mental phenomena occur due to the attempt to cope with hard problems. He also developed procedures such as free association and dream analysis for delving into one's conscious and unconscious parts of personality. These techniques are widely used in therapy today to treat many mental disorders. However, Freud's psychodynamic paradigm has been critiqued by many. A prominent criticism to Freud's stages of development is that no scientific data support any of the stages and much of his theorizing is based on case studies. His theories have also been criticized for their overemphasis on sex drive. Nevertheless, Freud's theory of development did open the doors for psychologists to develop theories on how a child develops and how childhood occurrences could lead to subsequent adult behavior. It was also the impetus of theories that describe the abnormal behaviors of individuals.

APPLICATION OF THE PSYCHOANALYTIC THEORY TO EATING BEHAVIOR

As Freud advocated through his concept of psychic determinism, every action we undertake is not an accident, but has a cause behind it. According to Freud, these causes reside in one's unconscious mind that is not directly accessible to us. Only through techniques such as free association, journaling, drawing, and talking it out can these causes become known to the individual. Regardless of the eating plan to which you are adhering, there will be instances where one will not adhere to it 100 percent of the time. To determine why these episodes occur, one needs to utilize the process of *introspection*, the self-observation and reporting of inner conscious thoughts, desires, and motives. This can be accomplished through the process of daily journaling. If one is diligent about recording one's thoughts and behaviors as they are occur, then they are available for objective evaluation by oneself and or a therapist to determine a cause-and-effect relationship.

Another aspect that Freud advocated, through his psychosexual stages of development, was how our childhood development can affect our later adult behavior. By conducting a research investigation into one's childhood and past, the origin of many of our maladaptive behaviors can be brought to light. A therapist can help guide one through the introspection process or one can conduct the fact-finding process through the help of family, relatives, old photographs, and videos. Through the process, one may find maladaptive behavioral patterns that were reinforced from early childhood (e.g., parents offering a sweet treat to the child each time the child became upset or got hurt). Once these "ah-ha" moments are illuminated, proactive alternative eating strategies can be developed.

Using defense mechanisms to help cope with difficult or painful situations is a common occurrence in life. However, our defenses mechanisms may thwart our efforts to accurately understand the problem at hand and heal or fix the problem. This is why it is imperative to identify the defense mechanisms that we utilize with regard to our eating behavior. By becoming familiar with the coping strategies that we employ for our eating behaviors, we will be on the path to positive change. The questionnaire on page 166 (**Figure 9–2**) should provide you with insight about your attitudes toward your weight and eating behavior, and more specifically the defense mechanisms that you typically employ.

Defense Mechanism Scale

Directions: Evaluate each statement by using the following scale.

5 = strongly disagree 4 = somewhat disagree, 3 = neutral, 2 = somewhat agree, 1 = strongly agree,

1. When trying on new clothing that is tight, I typically attribute it to clothing sizes running small. _____

2. I conclude that my older clothing is too small because it shrank in the laundry. _____

3. I try not to think about my weight or appearance as an issue. _____

Denial Score Total_____

Rationalization

1. Because I am paying for the meal and because it includes foods that I don't eat at home, I feel that it is okay to overeat when I dine out. _____

2. I feel that parties and other social engagements are special occasions at which most people overindulge on food. _____

3. I blame my weight on factors that are beyond my control such as heredity, body type, and low metabolism. _____

Rationalization Score Total _____

Projection

1. When I see other people eating, I tend to look critically at the type and quantity of food they are eating. _____

2. When I see other people who are overweight, I tend to look critically at how they are dressed. I think they would look more attractive if they were thinner. _____

3. I look at overweight people and think they may have a problem with weight. _____

Projection Score Total_____

Displacement

1. I am tired of hearing about the latest diet fad every time I turn on the television. _____

2. I really don't think I need to change just because "thin is in." _____

3. Because of my weight problem, I get angry with others. _____

Add your scores for each of the four scales.

Displacement Score Total_____

The highest score indicates your most relied upon defense mechanisms.

Insight

List your defenses in order from your highest to lowest scoring.

1. _____

2. _____

3. _____

4. _____

Source: Scale adapted from Dweck, J. (2004). *The Weight Loss Buddy®Losing for Good: How to Lose Weight and Help a Friend(s) Lose Weight.* Tenafly, NJ: Weight Loss Buddy Press.

Analyzing Your Results

➤ When looking over your results, you may see that you use more than one defense mechanism with regard to your eating behavior.

➤ Take some time to observe how often you rely on your defense mechanisms each day.

➤ Make a list of some of the situations that trigger your use of each of the defense mechanisms.

➤ Are there certain people in your life who trigger you to rely upon a specific defense mechanism? List these people for your reference.

➤ List some of the positive outcomes for using each one of your defenses.

➤ Now list some of the negative outcomes for using each one of your defenses.

➤ Ask yourself: "Are there more negative than positive outcomes?"

➤ Are you ready to develop some healthy alternative strategies to replace these defense mechanisms?

Healthy Strategies

You have now gained the insight about which defense mechanisms you use to distance yourself from the discomfort of acknowledging your eating and weight issues. In addition, you are now cognizant of some of the situations and individuals who trigger the use of these coping strategies. Now we will embark on counteracting these defense mechanisms that cloud our true thoughts.

➤ Start off envisioning a good friend of yours using these defense mechanisms instead of yourself. What would you recommend for him or her to do or think instead?

➤ Realize that you have been placing the blame elsewhere for your eating behavior. Though it is important to take responsibility for our actions, balance owning up to your behavior with a plan of change. In other words, balance the negative feelings of taking ownership with the positive feelings of enacting change.

➤ The more that you consistently counteract each of your defense mechanisms, the more comfortable you will feel with acknowledging the truth of your eating behavior. This may be an uncomfortable process in the beginning.

➤ For the denial defense mechanism, ask yourself to make a gentle "internal/dispositional attribution" for that situation instead of the "situational" ones that you typically make. Add a statement of positive self-talk to support changing that maladaptive eating pattern. For example, instead of saying to yourself "Eating these few slices of bread won't affect my gluten-free diet" (denial), it would be better to state "This bread smells good and looks good. If I eat it, I am choosing to suffer some serious consequences. I value my health more than the temporary satisfaction I would get from eating this bread. I have a strong sense of self control and choose not to eat it."

➤ If you typically engage in rationalization, then after you develop your rationalizing statement, attach a truly rational percentage to how likely you think that statement you made is typically true for the average person or situation. This strategy will help to put perspective on your rationalizing statements. For example, using the statement "If I don't eat this slice of Patty's cheesecake, she'd never forgive me," think about what percentage of people, put in the same situation, would think that this statement is true. Most likely, the percentage you assign to this statement would be very low. A true friend would forgive you for turning down a piece of their cheesecake so this statement is not very rational.

➤ As for individuals who use displacement as their primary defense, develop a variety of proactive ways that you could do to put that displaced anger or energy into good use (e.g., exercise, vigorous cleaning, gardening).

➤ Lastly, for persons who rely on projection: After projecting the critical blame to another, ask yourself honestly if that blame could be attributed to yourself as well.

➤ Don't get disheartened; this process of learning not to rely on defense mechanisms takes a great deal of time and practice for everyone.

Figure 9–2 Defense Mechanisms Scale.

Counteracting Your Dependence on Defense Mechanisms

Take some to time to reflect on your most frequently used defense mechanisms within the context of eating behavior. Consider using a journal to help you recognize the frequency with which you use a particular defense mechanism and the contexts in which you use it. Pay particular attention to the outcome (healthy or unhealthy eating behavior) that typically results. Many times simply being aware of the cause and effect relationship between a defense mechanism and unhealthy eating behavior can dramatically decrease your usage of the defense mechanism.

You might want to brainstorm and then include in your journal healthy alternative behaviors that would replace your reliance on a particular defense mechanism. For instance, if you typically rely on the displacement defense mechanism, and get angry at others when you overeat, turn that negative energy into something positive and exercise or vigorously garden. Each time that you use a healthy behavioral alternative, note it in your journal and the type of eating behavior that resulted (healthy or unhealthy). By reflecting several times a day on your journal and the healthy eating behavior that results from relying less on defense mechanism, you will start to see yourself making more healthy eating choices.

You Diagnose It

ADHERENCE SCENARIO 1

About 2 months ago, Regina and her fellow employees had to take a pay cut at their job so that their boss could make the payroll. In addition, Regina and her coworkers' workload increased. Regina is very unhappy about the situation and anxious about being able to pay her own bills. After work each day, Regina comes home and devours an entire box of cookies or a bag of potato chips, before facing her children and making dinner. When her husband asked her if she was upset, she adamantly stated "no." Now, Regina no longer heads for the kitchen when she comes home, but instead heads for her husband and finds something to criticize him about.

1. By using the psychoanalytic paradigm, discuss which two defense mechanisms Regina is engaging in.
2. What methods would a psychoanalyst suggest that Regina use to understand her eating behavior?

ADHERENCE SCENARIO 2

Reuben is a chef at the Plantation Restaurant. Since being hired at this job 2 years ago, Reuben has gained 19 pounds and has not adhered to the eating plan that his physician laid out for him. At his annual physical, his doctor is troubled by Reuben's weight gain and asks him why he is having trouble adhering to his eating plan.

1. Give a response that would indicate that Reuben is using the defense mechanism of repression.
2. Give a response that would indicate that Reuben is using the defense mechanism of sublimation.

Review

- ✓ Psychoanalysis is a group of theories developed by Austrian physician Sigmund Freud and further developed by other researchers.
- ✓ Psychic determinism is the assumption that everything a person thinks or does has a specific cause; most of the time, this cause can be found in the mental processes that are hidden in one's unconscious.
- ✓ Psychoanalytic theory revolves around the concept of psychic conflict or the tension between the id and the superego that the ego is moderating.
- ✓ According to Freud, all behavior is motivated by the desire to feel pleasure.
- ✓ Freud developed dynamic and psychosocial explanations for human behavior. He conceptualized the psychosexual stages of development. Freud believed that there are prominent stages in which an individual has a specific need, and if his or her needs are left unmet or overstimulated, there are lasting effects on an individual's behavior. Freud believed that the negative outcomes of each of these stages accounted for an individual's deviance or abnormal behavior. The five psychosexual stages are the oral stage, the anal stage, the phallic stage, the latency stage, and the genital stage.
- ✓ The ego uses what Freud calls defense mechanisms to keep forbidden impulses and disturbing thoughts suppressed in the unconscious mind.
- ✓ Defense mechanisms do not consistently keep forbidden impulses suppressed out of awareness because sometimes they "leak" into our conscious thoughts or behaviors in the form of parapraxes or Freudian slips.

D.I.E.T. (Do I Eat This?)

TIPS TO CONSIDER WHEN REACHING FOR A PIECE OF FOOD

- Am I using eating to express the emotions that I am feeling?
- Am I eating simply for the sake of a pleasure sensation or is it physical hunger?
- What would my superego or conscience say about me eating this type of food?
- If I put this piece of food down and instead talked about how I am feeling, would I still feel hungry?

REFERENCES

1. Brenner, C. (1974). *An Elementary Textbook of Psychoanalysis.* Garden City, NY: Doubleday/Anchor.
2. Kihlstrom, J.F. (1990). The psychological unconscious. In L. Pervin (Ed.), *Handbook of Personality: Theory and Research* (pp. 445–464). New York: Guilford.
3. Bornstein, R.F. (1999). Source amnesia, misattribution, and the power of unconscious perceptions and memories. *Psychoanalytic Psychology, 16,* 155–178.
4. Shaver, P.R., & Mikulincer, M. (2005). Attachment theory and research: Resurrection of the psychodynamic approach to personality. *Journal of Research in Personality, 39,* 22–45.
5. Brenner, C. (1974). *An Elementary Textbook of Psychoanalysis.* Garden City, NY: Doubleday/Anchor.
6. Gazzaniga, M.S., Ivry, R.B., & Mangun, G.R. (1998). *Cognitive Neuroscience: The Biology of the Mind.* New York: Norton.
7. Shaver, P.R., & Mikulincer, M. (2005). Attachment theory and research: Resurrection of the psychodynamic approach to personality. *Journal of Research in Personality, 39,* 22–45.
8. Suls, J., & Fletcher, B. (1985). The relative efficacy of avoidant and nonavoidant coping strategies. A meta-analysis. *Health Psychology, 4,* 249–288.
9. Baumeister, R.F., Dale, K., & Sommer, K.L. (1988). Freudian defense mechanisms and empirical findings in modern social psychology: Reaction formation, projection, displacement, undoing, isolation, sublimation, and denial. *Journal of Personality, 66,* 1081–1124.
10. Freud Is Not Dead. *Newsweek* (March 27, 2006)

CROSS-CULTURAL PERSPECTIVE

Chapter 10

Cross-Cultural Differences and Eating Behavior

LEARNING OBJECTIVES

By the end of this chapter, the reader will be able to:

1. Understand the value of examining eating behavior from a cross-cultural perspective.

2. Identify complex and tight cultures and how those characteristics influence our eating behavior.

3. Distinguish between collectivist and individualistic tendencies and how those traits foster eating behavior.

4. Apply strategies that will counteract cultural norms that facilitate maladaptive eating patterns.

Culture's Role in Indulgence

It was the Roman culture that was most famous for their fantastic feasting. Saturnalia was a public feast and festival in Rome, initiated around 217 BCE to raise citizen morale after a crushing military defeat.[1] Originally, it was celebrated for a day, on December 17, but its popularity caused it to grow into a weeklong feast, ending on the 23rd. Efforts to shorten the feast and celebration were unsuccessful. This was the first documented feast initiated where people were encouraged to eat to raise their woes. One could even go so far as to say that the Roman culture initiated emotion-based eating habits.

Feasts during medieval times would include elaborate diversions called *subtleties*, which were provided between each course. Servants would wheel in mechanical elephants, ships, and castles, and troubadours provided music and stories while spectacular fireworks lit up the skies. Sometimes entertainment appeared in the form of huge pies. In 1484, a huge pie made for the Duke of Burgundy's Feast of the Pheasant contained an entire group of musicians.[2]

Through the centuries traditions may change, but the human urge to feast will probably not go away because there are so many cultural reasons (e.g., to celebrate or to mourn) to gather with others and indulge. The feast gives all a moment of reprieve from one's life.

PSYCHOLOGY AND CULTURE

Culture refers to psychological characteristics of groups which include customs, beliefs, habits, and values that shape one's emotions, behaviors, and life patterns.[3] All aspects from one's culture such as language or a perception of reality are learned and are not innate. The process of picking up a new culture when one moves into a new country is called *acculturation*; a child upon being born, however, picks up his or her new culture through the process of *enculturation*. The concept of a cultural group is a difficult notion to wrap one's mind around because any group of people who are psychologically different from another group could potentially be termed as a cultural group. Historically, cultural groups are ethnic and linguistic, but prominent cultural distinctions can be identified within national and linguistic borders as well as across them. What makes the study of cultural groups even more challenging is that the psychologists who study cultures come from their own cultural groups that color the way that they see the world.

Cultures can be categorized and compared in several ways with regard to personality and emotions and how they shape their members' behaviors. Surprisingly, only in recent history have psychologists such as David McClelland begun to study human behavior with regard to cultural differences and similarities.[4] McClelland categorized cultures based upon their need for love and affiliation versus their need for high achievement. By looking at the stories that people in different cultures pass to their children (such as in the United States, *The Little Engine that Could*), McClelland discovered a trend. McClelland's research indicated that cultures that passed along stories that emphasized high achievement were likely to be cultures that showed greater rapid technological growth than cultures that passed along stories to their children emphasizing peace, harmony, and love.

Triandis followed up on McClelland's work and proposed that cultures vary with regard to three basic dimensions: complexity, tightness versus looseness, and collectivism versus individualism.[5,6] Complexity refers to how complicated a culture is, with modern, technologically advanced cultures generally being more complex than hunter/gatherer cultures. The tightness versus looseness dimensions are aimed at the level of deviation away from proper behavior that a culture tolerates. Cultures that tolerate only small deviations from cultural behaviors are referred to as tight cultures and cultures that allow large deviations from proper behavior are termed as loose cultures.

The last cultural dimension that Triandis proposed is collectivism versus individualism. These two dimensions are based on the way a culture views the relationship between the individual and society. Japan is considered a collectivist culture because the needs of the groups or of the "collective" are more important than the needs and rights of the individual, whereas, in individualist cultures like the United States, the individual and his or her choices are viewed as more important.[7] Prototypical collectivist cultures include Japan, China, and India, while prototypical individualistic cultures include the United States, Australia, Britain, Canada, and the Netherlands.[8] Within the United States, Hispanics, Asians, and African Americans are more collectivist than Anglos[9]; too, within the United States, women are typically more collectivist oriented than men.[10]

Markus and Kitayama report some interesting emotional differences between individualist and collectivist cultures. People in collectivist countries are more likely to feel other-oriented emotions such as sympathy and empathy, while people in individualist countries report feeling self-focused emotions such as anger more frequently. Also, individuals from collectivist-oriented countries seem to base their self-worth on fitting in socially with a group while individualist-oriented individuals base their self-worth on personal accomplishments.[11]

EATING HABITS

Eating habits refer to an entire host of concepts such as why and how people eat, the foods they choose to eat, with whom they eat, and the ways people obtain, store, use, and discard food. Individual, social, cultural, religious, economic, environmental, and political factors all influence people's eating habits. Humans' main motive to eat is to survive. Humans, though, also eat to show appreciation, for a sense of belonging, and as part of family traditions. For instance, someone who is not hungry might eat a sweet treat that has been baked in his or her honor.

LEARNED EATING BEHAVIORS

People eat according to their culture's learned behaviors regarding etiquette, meal and snack patterns, acceptable foods, food combinations, and portion sizes.[12] For instance, in some cultural groups, it is acceptable to lick one's fingers during eating, though for other groups, this is considered rude behavior. These eating rituals can be dependent on whether the meal is informal, formal, or special (e.g., birthday or holiday). Keep in mind that a *meal* is typically defined as the consumption of two or more foods in a structured setting at a specific time. Meals vary across cultures, but typically include grains like rice or noodles, meat or a meat substitute like fish, beans, or tofu, and side dishes such as vegetables. Civilized cultures around the world demand that meals shall be eaten with respect for the food and also for the people in whose company it is eaten. Humans usually eat in the company of others. Since eating typically happens more than once a day, humans turn meals into a time to learn and to practice their "culture." Politeness at meals then becomes second nature to those who take their meals in the presence of others. Eating rules or etiquette exist mainly to ensure that meals shall be shared peacefully.[13] Our ancestors killed and chopped their food prior to the meal. With knives and guns in their hands, hunger, and possibly alcohol in their systems, violence was evitable. Therefore, mealtime rules provide not only safety but also predictability that allows eaters to relax. Dining rules insist on no pointing with knives, forks, or spoons. Diners should not stab their food on their knives to carry it to their mouths or hold their knives in their fists and only lay down their blades facing inward not toward their neighbors.

Interestingly, the Chinese and Japanese have banned knives from the table altogether. The Chinese and Japanese usually cut up everything prior to the meal, far away and out of sight, and the diners are provided with blunt sticks as their eating utensils. People who use chopsticks eat quickly because the cut-up food is very hot and could get cold if too much time is taken up chatting rather than eating. Usually talking tends to be done before or afterward the meal in these cultures.

In the Western cultures, the majority of diners use forks as their utensil of choice. Eating with one's hands is permissible only for specific instances such as eating artichokes, corn on the cob or on informal occasions. There are also some rules of etiquette that most all cultures embrace, for practical reasons, such as "When eating refrain from speaking, lest the windpipe open before the gullet and life be in danger" (from the Babylonian Talmud, c. 450 CE).[14]

Another learned eating behavior in most of Europe and the Americas is that meals are eaten around a table, which signals the oneness of the group. However, the separateness and self-sufficiency of each individual is emphasized in the manner that the cutlery is laid out like a fence surrounding each place. Each diner sits on his or her own upright chair and is served on a separate dish. Crossing over another diner's boundaries (e.g., sampling food from their plate) is generally taboo or demonstrates great intimacy between two people. Though in other cultures, there is no insistence on eating boundaries as diners take the food from a common focal point with their hands, while typically sitting on the ground. People who take their food from a central dish or set of dishes necessarily interact in the process, so they concentrate on eating with fairness and consideration and tend to talk little.

Hospitality, which is hosting nonfamily members in one's house, is another learned behavior that is the subject of rules and constraints. Hosts have to make guests "feel at home," while guests must refrain from making demands for different foods or from overstepping their boundaries. Hosts give, while guests receive. Due to this imbalance between hosts and guests, guests are to reciprocate back by expressing their appreciative attitudes toward the food and eating all that the host has served.[15,16]

Formal versus informal meals also bring with them an entire set of eating protocol. Formal meals are likely to be "feasts" on the occasion of events important for the community. People come together to eat when they wish to celebrate or mourn, especially when they are eager to express what is held in common.[17] *Formality* is, among other things, taking time to enjoy the meal and what it represents. Informal meals sometimes are not a source of leisurely pleasure, but can be something done purely out of necessity. The meal is eaten as quickly as possible to get it out of the way in favor of other activities. The act of preparing food is often eliminated entirely, and prepared food is substituted. Informal meals seem to be the growing trend in U.S. society with little thought going into the food-preparation and the consumption processes.

Food combinations and flavors is another area in which cultures differ from one another. A liking for some flavors or food combinations may come naturally, but others must be learned. The more a person is exposed to a certain food, the more the person becomes familiar and less fearful of the food, and may consume it more often. A cultural group often provides guidelines regarding acceptable foods, food combinations, eating patterns, and eating behaviors. Adherence to these guidelines creates a sense of identity and belonging for the individual. For instance, a prototypical U.S. meal consists of a hamburger, french fries, and a soda pop. Some individuals may consume these meals not for their nutritional benefits, but to give them a sense of belongingness.

RELIGIOUS DIETARY BEHAVIORS

Religious beliefs can influence a person's dietary practices, which can ultimately affect food selection. The level of commitment that an individual has toward their religion may determine if they adopt the dietary practices of that religion. An understanding of various religious beliefs as they relate to diet can help practitioners make recommendations for nutrition adherence plans.

Hinduism, common among persons of Indian descent, is the oldest religion in the world. Hindus respect all life forms, both human and animal. Because they represent life, meat or eggs are not consumed, nor are chicken and pigs, because these animals are considered scavengers. Most Hindus are vegetarians, but some eat fish and may consume dairy foods.

Buddhism is typically practiced by persons from Southeast Asia; more specifically, Vietnam, Cambodia, Laos, Tibet, China, Japan, and Thailand. There are many different sects of Buddhism and each sect may have established rules regarding food choices. Some sects promote vegan diets while others permit meat that is considered "pure meat," meaning the animal has died of natural causes. Other sects may consume fish or chicken, but no other type of animal flesh. Moderate eating, not indulging, is a typical practice for Buddhists and rice is a staple for most Buddhists.

Judaism can be traced back to the ancient Hebrews. Jewish dietary laws are biblical ordinances that include rules regarding food, chiefly about the selection, slaughter, and preparation of meat. Kosher food products, which are ritually prepared and approved for consumption, are designated with the appropriate mark such as K or U. Some protein and calorie supplements are kosher approved and also are identified by the K or U symbols on the label. The most devout members of the Jewish faith do not combine milk and meat in the same meal; traditional orthodox Jewish homes keep two sets of dishes, silver, and utensils: one for milk and one for meat. Healthcare institutions with a large Orthodox clientele have Orthodox kitchens, where separate utensils and dishes for meat and dairy foods are used. Many Jewish people, even those not strictly kosher, adhere to the rule to forsake consumption of all animals that do not have cloven hooves and do not chew their cud. Hence, most Jewish people do not consume pork and pork products. Also, any seafood that does not have fins and scales is forbidden. This means shellfish; lobsters, oysters, shrimp, clams, and crabs are not appropriate choices for this group.

Islam (Muslim) is the newest of the most prominent religions and is growing quickly. Muslims are advised to stop eating when they are still hungry and to always share food. The dietary laws developed by Muhammad prohibit eating swine and drinking alcohol. Saum, the ritual of fasting observed during the 30 days of Ramadan, requires not eating from sunrise until sunset. The sanctity or preserving of life is important to Muslims.

FOOD PATTERNS OF SPECIFIC POPULATIONS

The U.S. Census Bureau data indicate as of July 2006 approximately one in three U.S. residents (about 100 million people) was of minority heritage.[18] According to the data, the largest minority group is the Hispanics (44.3 million, 14.8 percent of the population), followed by black Americans (40.2 million or roughly 13.5 percent of the population) and then Asians (14.9 million). By 2050, the census bureau projects the non-white population to reach approximately 235.7 million or 54 percent of the U.S. population. The Hispanic population is projected to triple, and the Asian population is expected to double. Other populations such as American Indians and Alaskan natives also are projected to increase from 4.9 million to 8.6 million (or from 1.6 percent to 2 percent of the total population).

With these population changes, big variations in language, culture, religious beliefs, education, and food habits are expected within each minority group.

Hispanic Food Patterns

It is important to become familiar with the eating habits of each of these large minority groups. The U.S. Census Bureau categorizes the Hispanic/Latino profile as Cubans, Mexicans, Puerto Ricans, and South and Central Americans.[19] In the United States, Mexican Americans comprise 60 percent of the Hispanic/Latino population. Mexicans live predominantly in California, Texas, Arizona, New Mexico, and Colorado. The difference between Mexican, Puerto Rican, and other Latin American countries is 500 years of separate history, as well as entirely different native populations that were present when the Spaniards arrived. Thus, the Mexican, Puerto Rican, and Latin American cultures each have a completely different concept of what foods are acceptable and appropriate.

The Mexican Diet

Since there are so many categories in the Hispanic population, we will focus on the dietary behavior of just one population, the Mexicans. The Mexican diet today is rich in a variety of foods and dishes that comprise a blend of pre-Columbian, Spanish, French, and more recently, U.S. culture.[19] The typical Mexican diet is rich in complex carbohydrates, which come from corn and corn tortillas (although more flour tortillas are consumed in northern parts of Mexico and here in the United States), pinto and black beans, Spanish rice, and Mexican sweet bread. The typical Mexican diet contains an adequate amount of protein in the forms of beans, eggs, fish, and shellfish, and a variety of meats, including beef, pork, poultry and goat.

Because frying is the typical cooking method, the Mexican diet is also high in fat. Popular vegetables in the traditional diet are cactus (nopales), onions, peas, squash, and tomatoes. Vegetables that are commonly missing from the diet include dark-green leafy and deep-yellow vegetables, foods that many Hispanics are not familiar with. Fruits include semitropical and tropical fruits such as bananas, mangos, guavas, papayas, and pineapples, which are often eaten as snacks.

Traditional Beliefs

Some Hispanics of various cultures believe in the "hot" and "cold" concept of foods, herbs, and illnesses. As part of this belief, a good meal provides a balance of hot and cold foods and those who eat foods with temperatures that are wrong for them can get sick. "Hot" foods include chili peppers, garlic, onions, most grains, expensive cuts of meat, oils, and alcohol. "Cold" foods are most vegetables, tropical fruits, dairy products, and inexpensive cuts of meat.

Traditionally, Mexicans ate four or five meals daily. The foods eaten vary with factors such as income, education, urbanization, geographic region, and family customs. The extent to which the traditional Mexican meal pattern continues among Mexicans in the United States has not been closely studied, but the three-meal pattern typically prevails. The daily meal pattern in the typical Mexican American home varies according to the availability of traditional foods and the degree of assimilation into U.S. society.

Emigration Changes

With emigration to the United States, prominent changes resulted in the Mexican American's diet. Healthy changes occurred such as a moderate increase in the consumption of milk, vegetables, and fruits, and a large decrease in the consumption of lard and cream. The introduction of salads and cooked vegetables has increased the use of fats, such as salad dressings and butter. Another less-healthy change is the strong decline in the consumption of fruit-based beverages in favor of high-sugar drinks. Consumption of inexpensive sources of carbohydrates, like beans and rice, also has decreased as a result of acculturation.

The Hispanic Lifestyle

The family unit is the single most important social unit in the life of Hispanics. Family responsibilities come before all other responsibilities. Gender differentiation and male dominance are issues to consider while working with Hispanic families. The father is the leader of the family, and the mother runs the household, shops, and prepares the food. The traditional concepts of manhood and womanhood, however, appear to be changing toward a more egalitarian model with increased exposure to U.S. society.

The healthcare advisor may intervene with Hispanic clients and communities in culturally sensitive ways, which includes viewing culture as a boon rather than a resistant force, incorporating cultural beliefs into care plans, stressing familianism, and taking time for conversation.

Asian Food Patterns

The classification of Asians from the U.S. Census Bureau includes persons from a wide variety of countries, including Vietnam, China, India, Pakistan, and Japan. People from these cultures have diverse food habits, though meal composition and cooking processes are similar across Asian regions. Food preparation techniques include stir-frying, barbecuing, boiling, and steaming.[20] These cooking techniques may prevent losing important nutrients. An additional common theme is that dairy products are rarely used by this population. Most Asian cultures get their protein from fish, pork, and poultry, which can provide adequate amounts if food intake is sufficient. The major staple in all of the diets in this culture is rice, including products made with rice flour, which provides energy. Vegetables and fruits are also a prominent part of the diet for Asians. Focusing only on the traditional Chinese diet, we find that more than 80 percent of its calories come from grains, legumes, and vegetables and 20 percent from animal protein, fruits, and fats.[21] Interestingly, most Asians are lactose intolerant and obtain calcium from processed tofu which utilizes calcium sulfate in the manufacturing process.[22] Soybeans and fresh tofu are naturally low in calcium. Other foods that are consumed as good sources of calcium include the bones of small fish and dark green, leafy vegetables.

Another food issue that is related to the Chinese culture is the need for a balance between yin and yang and among the five elements of water, fire, earth, metal, and wood. Yin foods are hot, higher in calories (e.g. milk, honey, sugar) and believed to increase circulation by raising the metabolism; yang foods are cool and eliminate toxins by decreasing the metabolism (e.g. eggs, meat, fish, cheese). The optimal Chinese diet is comprised of a blend of both types of food to keep the body balanced. Traditionally, the less active the person, the more yin food that is required.

African American Food Patterns

Research indicates that today's prototypical African American diet is influenced by the lifestyle of the ancestors who lived in the southern United States.

The traditional African American diet consists of pork and chicken that is fried, boiled, stewed, or barbequed; catfish; legumes; rice; potatoes; grits; collard greens; and other dark-green and yellow vegetables. This diet is high in vitamin A, iron, and fiber. In the African American culture, the food is often fried and covered with heavy sauces and gravies that increase the fat and caloric content of meals. Similarly, many African Americans are lactose intolerant and, as a result, might not consume much milk or cheese.

The food habits of today's African Americans are more likely to reflect the family's economic status, where they live, and their work schedules. Due to time constraints, traditional foods may only prepared on special occasions or holidays. Breakfast meals are much lighter than traditional breakfast meals and lunch often consists of fast food from a local restaurant. The dinner meal may include one or more traditional dishes, however, time constraints may prevent the usual preparation methods. For example, instead of cleaning, chopping, and boiling collard greens with ham hocks, boiled green beans will be served.

HEALTH CONCERNS OF MINORITY POPULATIONS

Data from the 2007 Behavioral Risk Factor Surveillance System (BRFSS) indicate that the rate of obesity in the United States was 25.6 percent in 2007.[23] Ethnic groups, such as Mexican Americans and African Americans, have higher rates of obesity and diabetes than other population groups. Research suggests that Hispanics are twice as likely to have diabetes as non-Hispanics, while African American adults are 1.9 times more likely than non-Hispanic white adults to have diabetes.

Research has reported a high prevalence of obesity, cardiovascular disease, diabetes, and dental cavities in the Mexican American population. Research studies also indicate that Mexicans in the United States eat more meat and saturated fats than Anglos and use fewer low-fat dairy products. Mexicans also are less likely to recognize high-fat foods. Approximately 10 to 12 percent of Mexican American adults have diabetes, with 95 percent of those having the noninsulin-dependent type.[24]

APPLYING KNOWLEDGE OF CULTURAL ISSUES TO NUTRITION ADHERENCE

With these statistics in mind, let's take our knowledge of cultural differences and apply psychological strategies to counteract these maladaptive eating behaviors.

Intake Techniques

When healthcare providers evaluate individuals from another culture, the intake-assessment process should include questions concerning their beliefs and the strength of them with regard to their cultural system. The ABCDE (Attitudes, Beliefs, Content, Decision Making, and client's Environment) interview technique should be used in the intake process to ferret out important cultural information that could affect the client's adherence to their prescribed eating plan.[25] By incorporating the client's cultural values into his or her eating plan, the likelihood that the client will adhere to the plan is much higher than if these values were ignored. However, maladaptive dietary cultural practices (e.g., deep-frying food, consistent informal meals on the run) should be acknowledged by the healthcare provider and healthy alternatives suggested.

When interviewing patients and/or families, it is important to keep in mind differences in communication styles between U.S./Western and non-Western cultures. For instance, eye contact is esteemed by Caucasian Americans but is considered impolite for many Asian and Native Americans. Greeting on a first-name basis indicates disrespect in some cultures. After finishing a nutrition assessment, the healthcare provider compares the client's nutrient needs to their current food intake. They then develop an eating plan that is respectful of that individual's cultural values, but also considers their specific medical condition and dietary constraints.

The ABCDE Cultural Food Interview Technique

A = Cultural-based Attitudes of clients and families
toward food
B = Beliefs: religious beliefs, food rituals, and traditions
C = Content: personal history, including economics, emigration,
and the role of food in the family
D = Decision-making style within the family and culture
E = Environment: the extent to which the client adheres to his or her
cultural norms

ATTITUDES

The following are some areas that a healthcare provider might want to consider with regard to the cultural-based attitudes that the client has toward food.

Questions to ask the client:

1. How are meals and snacks viewed in your household, neighborhood, community, and/or country? As a necessity which one needs to partake in quickly so one can get on to other activities? As a chance to catch up with other family members and friends? As a time for relaxation? (These questions are an opportunity for the healthcare provider to assess the client's sense of individualism versus collectivism.)

Note: If a client's attitude is discrepant with regard to a healthy eating plan, the healthcare advisor can use the central or the peripheral route of persuasion to change the client's attitude toward meals so that it is consistent with a healthy eating plan.

2. How much thought and planning do you and your family or friends put into making a meal or snack? Does a great deal of forethought go into making sure that the meal is nutritionally balanced? Do you consider making sure that old family recipes or meals from your heritage are made often?

3. How important is it to you that you eat foods from your cultural heritage?

4. Which cooking technique do you rely on most to cook your meals (e.g., frying, baking, boiling, steaming)? Is this technique learned from family members or your heritage?

BELIEFS

The following are some areas that a healthcare provider might want to consider with regard to the cultural-based beliefs that the client has toward food.

Questions to ask the client:

1. Do you adhere to any type of religious dietary restrictions or rituals? If yes, elaborate on these.

2. Are your meals informal or formal?

3. Where in your home do you eat your meals and/or snacks (e.g., dining room table, living room in front of the TV, or at the bar counter)?

4. How many minutes does each meal generally take you to consume?

5. What type of etiquette or rules do you and your family members follow at each of your meals (e.g., napkin on lap, use of utensils, prayer)?

CONTENT

The following are some areas that a healthcare provider might want to consider with regard to how the client's personal cultural history affects their eating behavior.

Questions to ask the client:

1. To what extent do food prices influence the types of foods that you purchase? Are there some foods that you would like to purchase or purchase more often, but due to economic circumstances you cannot?
2. Have your eating patterns changed throughout your life thus far? If so, how?
3. What eating patterns do you embrace that your family and relatives follow? Do you feel obligated to adopt these eating patterns because of pressure from family members or was it based upon your own choice? (Be mindful of assessing collectivist versus individualistic characteristics.)
4. Did you immigrate to this country? If so, are there foods from your homeland that you like to consume but cannot find now? Do you use the same cooking techniques that you used in your homeland?

DECISION-MAKING STYLE

The following are some areas that a healthcare provider might want to consider with regard to the client's decision-making style toward eating choices.

Questions to ask the client:

1. Who in your family is responsible for the grocery shopping and choosing the foods to purchase? Is this a shared responsibility?
2. Who in your family is responsible for cooking the majority of the meals?
3. To what extent do you have a role in choosing the types of foods that are served for each meal?
4. Are other family members given a chance to choose the meals that are served?

Note: If the healthcare advisor finds that the client engages in consistent collectivistic and strong normative eating practices (e.g., letting others choose one's foods, adopting eating behaviors because of familial pressure), then strategies to develop more individualistic characteristics and eating choices should be encouraged.

ENVIRONMENT

The following are some areas that a healthcare provider might want to consider with regard to the client's adherence to his or her cultural food norms.

Questions to ask the client:

1. To what extent do you feel it is important to pass down a sense of cultural tradition and heritage to your children or relatives?
2. Are there foods from other cultures that you integrate into your meals?
3. Is there a family member or friend who exerts influence over what you eat?
4. Do you feel comfortable eating foods from your culture at your workplace?

Cultural Diversity in the Food Industry

Cultural diversity in America is changing the healthcare and food service landscape. Assisted-living and long-term care facilities are now providing environments that are as homelike as possible. For patients in these facilities, healthcare providers should encourage family members to suggest culturally appropriate foods that the facility can provide. The facility also should encourage family members to provide familiar foods from home, especially if the patient's meal intake at the facility is poor. Familiar foods serve two main benefits: They make the care environment more homelike and also may encourage greater nutrition consumption.

Cultural diversity is a major issue in U.S. eating. To truly understand the impact cultures play in U.S. nutrition, one must examine both food and culture. Given the range of the variations that exist in each cultural group (i.e., socioeconomic status, religion, age, education, social class, location, length of time in the United States, and location of origin), caution needs to be taken not to generalize these characteristics to all individuals of a cultural group, but instead learn about each client and develop an eating plan sensitive to their cultural values and heritage, while discouraging or eliminating unhealthy eating practices.

Figures 10–1 and **10–2** illustrate the variance in food choices, food intake, and food expenditure over a 1-week time frame among various cultural groups. Look at the photos for similarities and differences between the cultural groups. Notice the number of persons in each household, their gender, and age. These are other factors to consider when looking at cultural diversity and food intake.

SUMMING IT UP

Knowing what culture a client is from can provide only limited information about the client's eating behaviors. As you have seen, there are numerous

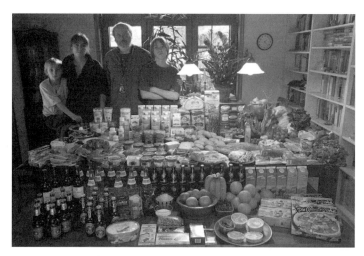

Figure 10–1 Germany: The Melander family of Bargteheide food expenditure for one week: 375.39 Euros or $500.07.

Source: © Peter Menzel/menzelphoto.com

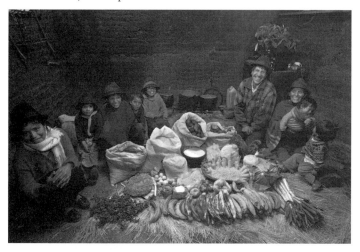

Figure 10–2 Ecuador: The Ayme family of Tingo food expenditure for one week: $31.55.

Source: © Peter Menzel/menzelphoto.com

other factors that need to be explored (e.g., adherence to cultural norms, diabetes, number of persons in the household) that can affect one's dietary choices. A culturally sensitive thorough and thoughtful intake process will provide a comprehensive portrait of the client's past and present eating behavior, so that the nutrition practitioner can develop an eating plan that his or her client will have the highest probability of adhering to.

You Diagnose It

ADHERENCE SCENARIO 1

Rosa has a very close extended family. Four nights a week, a different member of her extended family (e.g., aunt, cousin) hosts dinner at their home for everyone. For each dinner, usually 18 to 22 of Rosa's relatives are in attendance. Not only are the dinners seen as a time to catch up with the family members, but it is considered a time for the hosts to show off their culinary skills.

1. Rosa explains to her Registered Dietician that because of these dinners, she is not able to adhere to the eating plan her RD has prescribed. Rosa feels obligated to partake in every dinner and show her respect to the host by eating all of her meal. Give a cultural explanation for Rosa's nonadherence to her eating plan.
2. Discuss two situational factors that Rosa could control or change so that she will still be able to attend the dinners, but adhere to her eating plan.

ADHERENCE SCENARIO 2

Andrew and his wife just bought a 72-inch flat-screen TV. They are so enthusiastic about their new TV that they are eating their dinners in front of it each night on TV trays with paper plates. Prior to purchasing the TV, Andrew and his wife would enjoy a quiet candlelight dinner in the dining room, complete with linen napkins. Andrew has noticed that since acquiring the new TV, he has not been sticking to his regular exercise routine and has gained about 7 pounds.

1. Give a cultural explanation/eating habits explanation for Andrew's nonadherence behavior.
2. Discuss four situational changes that Andrew and his wife could make to promote adherence to a healthier food plan and better eating behaviors.

Review

- ✓ Culture refers to psychological characteristics of groups which include customs, beliefs, habits, and values that shape one's emotions, behaviors, and life patterns.
- ✓ The process of picking up a new culture when one moves into a new country is called acculturation; while a child, upon being born, picks up his or her new culture through the process of enculturation.

✓ Complexity refers to how complicated a culture is with modern, technologically advanced cultures generally more complex than hunter/ gatherer cultures. The tightness versus looseness dimensions are aimed at the level of deviation away from proper behavior that a culture tolerates.

✓ Collectivist cultures are focused on the needs of the groups or of the collective and they see these needs as more important than the needs and rights of the individual.

✓ In individualist cultures like the United States, the individual and his or her choices are viewed as more important.

✓ Eating habits refers to an entire host of concepts such as why and how people eat, the foods they choose to eat, with whom they eat, and the ways people obtain, store, use, and discard food. Individual, social, cultural, religious, economic, environmental, and political factors all influence people's eating habits.

✓ The ABCDE interview technique should be used in the intake process to ferret out important cultural information that could affect the client's adherence to their eating plan.

D.I.E.T. (Do I Eat This?)

TIPS TO CONSIDER WHEN REACHING FOR A PIECE OF FOOD

- Am I eating at a proper pace as my culture's etiquette dictates?
- Am I eating just to please the host?
- Am I engaging in proper eating decorum at the table?
- Am I only eating this type of food because it is what everyone in my culture eats?

REFERENCES

1. Kerrigan, M. (2001). *Ancient Rome and the Roman Empire.* London, UK: Dorling Kindersley.
2. Calmette, J., & Weightman, D. (1962). *The Golden Age of Burgundy: The Magnificent Dukes and Their Courts,* trans. New York: W.W. Norton.
3. Tseng, W.-S. (2003). *Clinician's Guide to Cultural Psychiatry.* San Diego: Academic Press.
4. McClelland, D.C. (1961). *The Achieving Society.* Princeton, NJ: Van Nostrand.
5. Triandis, H.C. (1994). *Culture and Social Behavior.* New York: McGraw-Hill.

6. Triandis, H.C. (1997). Cross-cultural perspectives on personality. In R. Hogan, J. Johnson, & S. Briggs (Eds.), *Handbook of Personality Psychology* (pp. 440–464). San Diego, CA. Academic Press.

7. Markus, H.R., & Kitayama, S. (1991). Culture and the self: Implications for cognition, emotion, and motivation. *Psychological Review, 98,* 224–253.

8. Hofstede, G. (1984). The cultural relativity of the quality of life concept. *Academy of Management Review, 9,* 389–398.

9. Triandis, H.C. (1994). *Culture and Social Behavior.* New York: McGraw-Hill.

10. Lykes, M.B. (1985). Gender and individualistic versus collectivist bases for notions about the self. In Lykes, M.B, & Stewart, A.J. (Eds.). (1985). *Gender and personality.* (pp. 269-295). Durham, NC: Duke University Press.

11. Markus, H.R., & Kitayama, S. (1991). Culture and the self: Implications for cognition, emotion, and motivation. *Psychological Review, 98,* 224–253.

12. Douglas, M., & Gross, J. (1981). Food and culture: Measuring the intricacy of rule systems. *Social Science Information 20,* 1–35.

13. Ibid.

14. Neusner, J. (1992). *Sources and Traditions: Types of Compositions in the Talmud of Babylonia.* Atlanta: Scholars Press.

15. Lévi-Strauss, C. (1969). The principle of reciprocity. (pp. 52–68) in R. Needham (Ed.) *The Elementary Structures of Kinship.* Oxford: Alden Press.

16. Pitt-Rivers, J. (1977). The law of hospitality. In J. Pitt-Rivers, *The Fate of Shechem or the politics of sex: Essays in the anthropology of the Mediterranean.* Cambridge, UK: Cambridge University Press.

17. Douglas, M., & Gross, J. (1981). Food and culture: Measuring the intricacy of rule systems. *Social Science Information 20,* 1–35.

18. U.S. Census Bureau. (2000). Minority population tops 100 million. Available at: www.census.gov/PressRelease/www/releases/archives/population/010048.html. Accessed December, 2009.

19. McWilliams, M. (2007). *Food Around the World: A Cultural Perspective.* Upper Saddle River, NJ: Pearson, 36–40.

20. Ibid.

21. Ibid.

22. Ibid.

23. Behavioral Risk Factor Surveillance System. (2007). Available at: www.cdc.gov/brfss. Accessed, December, 2009.

24. McWilliams, M. (2007). *Food Around the World: A Cultural Perspective.* Upper Saddle River, NJ: Pearson, 36–40.

25. Kagawa-Singer, M., & Blackhall, L. (2001). Negotiating cross-cultural issues at the end of life. *Journal of the American Medical Association, 286,* 2993–3001.

Section

VI

THE BIOLOGICAL PERSPECTIVE

Chapter 11

Biology and Eating Behavior

LEARNING OBJECTIVES

By the end of this chapter, the reader will be able to:

1. Understand the value of examining eating behavior from a biological perspective.

2. Become familiar with how specific regions of the brain, hormones, neurotransmitters, the thyroid, and genetics influence our eating behavior.

3. Apply strategies that will counteract biological influences that facilitate maladaptive eating patterns.

Is Your Brain's "Yum" Factor Sluggish?

"Did her brain get a hit of happiness after downing that milkshake?" That was the question that researchers at the Oregon Research Institute were assessing during their study of brain scans that was published in a 2008 issue of the journal of *Science*.[1]

Using a brain scanner, these scientists watched young women savor milkshakes. What they found was counterintuitive; overweight women did not receive a "hit" or the reinforcement of happiness in the dorsal striatum region of their brain after drinking their shake, but nonoverweight women did. Eric Stice and his research colleagues believe that when the brain doesn't sense enough gratification from food, people may overeat to compensate.

This innovative study can predict which individuals will pack on pounds during the next year because they may have a gene that make their brain's "yum" factor more sluggish than the average individual's.

Exercise and a balanced healthy diet help to manage one's weight, but scientists also know that genetics play a key role in obesity, in particular, the neurotransmitter dopamine, one of the prominent brain chemicals that senses pleasure. Though eating can temporarily boost dopamine levels, research indicates that obese individuals have fewer dopamine receptors in their brains than thin individuals. Additionally, the gene version, Taq1A1, is linked to fewer dopamine receptors.

A BRIEF HISTORY OF BIOPSYCHOLOGY

The last psychological perspective to be discussed is the biological perspective. In these last two chapters, we will explore the question "To what extent is our eating behavior a product of biological processes or reducible to the processes of the body and the brain?" The application of the principles of biology to the study of mental processes and behavior is referred to as biopsychology or neuropsychology.

The field of biological psychology has been around for almost a thousand years. Historians date this field back to a Persian psychologist and physician, Avicenna (980–1037), who noted in *The Canon of Medicine* that physiological psychology could be used in treating emotion-based illnesses.[2] He based this assumption on research he conducted on changes in pulse rate and inner emotions. After the field's early beginnings, philosophers in the 18th and 19th centuries, such as Rene Descartes, proposed theories on how specific regions of the brain affected animal and human behavior. William James, a philosopher who wrote one of the earliest textbooks on psychology *The Principles of Psychology* (1890), stated that the scientific study of psychology should be grounded in the concepts of biology.[3]

RESEARCH METHODS USED BY BIOPSYCHOLOGISTS

Biopsychologists use several unique research methodologies to test their hypotheses. One of the earliest techniques that researchers used to study the relationship between brain regions and resulting behavior was studying brain-damaged individuals. One of the most famous cases of study occurred in 1848, when a construction supervisor for the railroads, Phineas Gage, was the victim of a dynamite explosion. That explosion resulted in a three-and-a-half-foot iron rod being impaled through his left check, into the frontal lobes of his brain, and out the top of his head. Amazingly, Gage survived, and at first, all seemed intact, including as his memory and speaking ability. Later, Gage's physician reported that Gage's personality began to change substantially as he became fitful while manifesting frequent incidents of extreme profanity and expressing little patience and restraint.[4,5] Gage's skull was preserved and scientists for over a century have studied the relationship between the regions of his skull damage and the resulting behavior that was so carefully noted by his physician.

Another method that biopsychologists use to understand the relationship between the brain and our behavior is to create lesions. A *lesion* is a brain-region of interest that is destroyed or stimulated so that changes such as depredated or enhanced performance on some behavioral measure can be observed. The neural tissue of interest can be destroyed or temporarily disabled through various methods: the application of electrical shock, by the infusion of a neurotoxin, or by the use of anesthetics. When a biopsychologist wants to understand the effects of stimulating a specific region of the brain, he or she typically applies electrical stimulation to that region so that neural activity is enhanced by the application of a small electrical current. To measure the neural activity of that region or of a specific neuron(s), the researcher attaches electrodes to the scalp of the subject to record the firing activity of the neurons. Functional magnetic resonance imaging (fMRI) is another method to measure enhanced neural activity by recording the cerebral blood flow, which indicates the activity of larger portions of the brain. These changes in blood flow can be detected with an MRI apparatus.

RESEARCH FINDINGS

The following section will illustrate some of the more prominent research advances that have occurred in pinpointing which regions of the brain are responsible for various forms of eating behavior. These studies have built upon the previously discussed research methodologies.

Regions of the Brain and Eating Behavior

In 2008, Gene-Jack Wang and his colleagues at the U.S. Department of Energy's Brookhaven National Laboratory in New York found new clues to how the brain and the stomach interact with emotions to cause overeating and ultimately obesity.[6] Wang and his fellow researchers examined how the human brain responded to "fullness" signals sent to it by an implanted device that stimulated the stomach. The scientists pinpointed the brain circuits that motivate the desire to overeat in the obese. Interestingly, these same brain circuits are the ones that cause addicted individuals to crave drugs. Further, the scientists also confirmed that these circuits play a key role in eating behaviors linked to soothing negative emotions.

Wang and colleagues examined the brain metabolism of seven obese participants who had gastric stimulators implanted for 1 to 2 years. The implanted stimulator, similar to a pacemaker, provides low levels of electrical stimulation to the vagus nerve, causing the stomach to expand and produce peptides that send messages of fullness to the brain.

The stimulator has been shown to reduce the urge to eat. Wang's study gives direct evidence of which specific brain regions are involved in the satiety response. Each participant in the research study received two separate positron emission tomography (PET) brain scans within 2 weeks. In one PET scan, the gastric stimulator was on; the other scan was given with the stimulator off. However, the participants were not told whether their stimulator was on or off. Before the scans, subjects were injected with a radioactively labeled form of glucose, which the scanner could follow to monitor brain metabolism.

The brain images revealed that specific regions had higher metabolic activity during gastric stimulation (the "on" condition) versus when the stimulator was off. The particular regions of the brain were the right hippocampus, the right cerebellum, the right orbitofrontal cortex, and the right striatum.

The changes observed were particularly prominent in the hippocampus, where metabolism was 18 percent higher during gastric stimulation. The hippocampus is associated with emotional behaviors, learning and memory, and processing of sensory and motor impulses. In addition, the hippocampus also plays a part in the retention of memories related to prior drug experiences in drug-addicted individuals. This finding suggests that satiety memories in obese individuals might also be stimulated by hippocampal activation.

The research participants were also asked to answer a questionnaire at each brain scanning session, which measured three parts of eating behavior: cognitive restraint, uncontrolled eating, and emotional eating. The results from the questionnaire revealed correlations between eating behaviors and areas of the brain activated by the stimulator. When gastric stimulation was occurring, scores on a measure of self-described "emotional eating" were 21 percent lower in comparison to when the stimulator was off.

More recently, Wang and colleagues conducted a study to examine sex differences in emotional eating and its relation to specific regions of the brain.[7] Ultimately, Wang found through the brain imaging study that hungry women can't control their desire for food as well as hungry men can. Wang's research may explain why women are more likely to engage in emotional eating than men and why women are less likely than men to lose weight while dieting. Wang believes that women have a much stronger reaction to food and it is harder to disengage that part of the brain that controls hunger perception and the desire to eat.

In his study, Wang tested 13 women and 10 men using PET brain scans. To ensure that the participants were hungry, the participants fasted for 18 hours before the scanning began. To tempt the participants, Wang had all of the participants' favorite foods on hand. This was so that researchers could examine what happens in the brain when a hungry person has the opportunity to see, taste (a small portion on a cotton swab), and smell their favorite foods, but not to eat them. The research participants did not get to eat until the 30-minute scans were finished and until after they completed a quiz on their feelings of hunger and desire for the food. Prior to their second set of scans, participants were told to practice ignoring the food. During this portion of scanning, they were told "to inhibit their desire for food and suppress their feelings of hunger."[8] The findings indicate that the male participants were fairly successful at this suppression because their brain scans showed much less hunger-related activity. However, as a group, the women were not as successful at suppressing their feelings of hunger as evidenced by extensive hunger-related activity shown in their brain scans.

Hormones and Eating Behavior

The question now is why did men's and women's brains respond differently in Wang and his colleague's study? Wang and his colleagues suspect that the difference is due to sex hormones, the chemical messengers that relay information through the bloodstream to other cells. Links have been found between female hormones and weight gain because some women tend to engage in binge eating in synchronization with their menstrual cycles. Pregnancy is another example where most women tend to overeat. Wang believes that women possibly have evolved to seek food more vigorously than their male counterparts. Due to women's instinct to reproduce and carry a baby, it is extremely imperative that they have constant food to support the reproductive process. In modern, developed societies, the avid seeking of food is no longer necessary for women, however, the brain-circuited behavior still remains.

Leptin

Another hormone, leptin, has been pinpointed as one of the key hormones that is responsible for reducing hunger, increasing the feeling of fullness, and controlling our fondness for food. Dr. Sadaf Farooqi and colleagues found that the pleasing properties of food have strong effects on the same key brain regions responsible for rewarding emotions and desires.[9] The researchers showed images of appetizing foods to participants who were deficient in the hormone leptin and measured which regions of their brains "lit up" as shown by using fMRI brain imaging. The pattern of brain activation after viewing the pictures of food was compared to the response after viewing pictures of non-food items like trees, cars, and boats. The patients who were lacking leptin had the striatal regions (similar to Wang's 2008 results) of their brain light up in response to pictures of food. These areas have been linked to pleasant and rewarding emotions and desires. When those patients were treated with leptin, responses to food pictures in these areas were reduced. In the control condition with participants who were not deficient in leptin, the striatal regions only lit up if the participants were hungry due to an overnight fast.

These findings have important ramification for the understanding of how two prominent systems, the pathways that control hunger and fullness and the brain processes involved in liking and wanting foods, interact. The researchers have clearly determined that hunger has an impact on activation in striatal regions of the brain in response to food pictures and the consumption of food modifies these responses. This modification requires the presence of the hormone leptin since, when it is deficient, these brain regions remain very sensitive to the presence and type of food pictures even after a meal.

Oxytocin

Research by Amico, Morris, and Vollmer have found that animals deficient in the hormone oxytocin are more likely to develop a sweet tooth.[10] *Oxytocin* is a hormone that plays a key role in physical and emotional responses because it induces labor, encourages maternal behavior, and promotes positive relationship interactions. In the study, Amico and colleagues compared two groups of mice (normal animals and those mice without the ability to produce oxytocin) to determine if they preferred drinking solutions with either added sugar or fat. The oxytocin-deficient mice showed significantly greater intake of the sugar solution than their control group counterparts, though both groups seemed to like the fat-enhanced drink just the same. This research sheds a new light on oxytocin in influencing food tastes and limiting intake of sweets. It has yet to be determined the extent that oxytocin plays in humans, but as far as the animal model is concerned, this craving for sweets is not considered a true eating disorder but that of a hormonal imbalance caused by lack of healthy nutrition.

TSH

The last hormone to be discussed that is linked to eating behavior is TSH, the thyroid-stimulating hormone produced in the butterfly-shaped thyroid gland which is located in the lower front of the neck. This hormone goes into the bloodstream where it helps the body to use energy, stay warm, and function properly. It's long been known that a very overactive thyroid can be linked to weight loss and a very underactive thyroid is associated with weight gain. Research by Fox and her colleagues, however, indicates that even variations within the normal range of thyroid function are related to weight changes.[11] The researchers examined the thyroid functioning of more than 2,400 men and women by looking at the results of their TSH tests. Fox and fellow colleagues found that variations, even small ones, over a period of several years in the participants' lives produced either weight loss or weight gain in both women and men alike. These findings suggest that physicians should monitor carefully the history of changes in their patients' TSH tests as potential moderators of weight gain or loss.

Neurotransmitters and Eating Behavior

Neurotransmitters, which are chemicals that relay, amplify, and modulate signals between a neuron and another cell, have also been found to affect eating behavior. Studies of neurotransmitter activity in the brain nerve cells have helped researchers learn more about disturbances of appetite, weight, and behavior. Many people who have eating disorders also have problems with depression, anxiety, and obsessions. Researchers have examined the association between depression, anxiety, and abnormal eating patterns to see if these problems represent some change in the activity of certain chemicals in the brain. Neurotransmitters that have been found to be of particular importance are serotonin and dopamine. These neurotransmitters have been associated with the control of hunger as well as depression, anxiety, obsessions, physical activity, and reward. Dopamine is the primary neurotransmitter involved in the reward pathways in the brain. Food intake is associated with dopamine release and feeling pleasure upon consumption. Evidence shows that obese individuals versus their lean counterparts have fewer dopamine (D2) receptors in the brain; it is thought that obese individuals overeat to compensate for this reward deficit. People with fewer of the dopamine receptors need to take in more of a rewarding/pleasurable substance, such as food or mood altering drugs, to get an effect that other people get with less.

Dopamine and Eating Disorders

Studies have suggested dopamine may play a role in anorexia and bulimia nervosa. Through PET imaging, Kaye and associates have shown that individuals with anorexia nervosa don't seek or respond to the types of pleasures most of us enjoy, including food.[12] These individuals also resist and ignore feedback that signals their ill state of health. Dr. Kaye and colleagues believes that an overactive dopamine receptor system in the antero-ventral striatum makes one vulnerable to these types of behaviors that signal symptoms of anorexia.

Kaye et al. (2005) in a different study found that the 10 women with a history of anorexia who, regardless of their age, body mass index, or time since recovery, exhibited overactive receptor systems in an area of the basal ganglia.[13] The amount of receptor activity was significantly greater than that of the 12 healthy women who were studied in the control group. The area affected was the antero-ventral striatum which contributes to how the brain responds to reinforcing experiences.

Other studies have shown this area also may have a role in addiction. In addition, many studies have shown that the dopamine system plays a key role in physical activity, and thus may help understand why people with anorexia nervosa often relentlessly exercise.

Genetics and Eating Behavior

The new field of nutrigenetics studies the genetic influences on what we eat as well as how much we eat and even our eating behavior. Nutrigenomics, another buzzword in the field, refers to the influence of diet on genes, mainly related to health and disease states such as obesity, cancer, and heart disease.

The fact that genes influence our taste perception is not a startlingly new discovery. The discovery of genetic variations in taste dates goes back to the 1930s when a chemist trying to develop a very bitter compound called phenylthiocarbamide (PTC) accidentally released some crystals into the air.[14] Interestingly, he found that some of his lab partners could barely stand the bitterness while others, himself included, hardly sensed anything. This finding spurred him to divide people into two groups: nontasters (or those with taste blindness) and tasters; thus, the science of taste genetics was started.

Though factors such as when we eat, what we eat, and how much we eat are largely determined by our culture, ethnic background, religion, and individual experiences, we now know that the interactions of genes plays just as prominent a role as environmental factors. In 2006, scientists working at the Monell Chemical Senses Center in Philadelphia found that the bitter taste gene receptor hTAS2R38 detects glucosinolates, a class of bitter compounds naturally found in various fruits and vegetables, especially varieties like broccoli, watercress, kale, bok choy, and turnips.[15]

The researchers tested bitterness ratings of these vegetables in 35 healthy adult participants expressing the three genotypes of hTAS2R38: PAV/PAV, PAV/AVI, and AVI/AVI (labeled after the three variable amino acids).

Typically, people with PAV/PAV are considered supertasters. These people are extremely sensitive to bitter tastes in foods such as coffee, tea, grapefruit juice, and vegetables and in manmade compounds such as PTC and 6-n-propylthiouracil (PROP), generally used in research. People with PAV from one parent and AVI from the other parent are medium tasters; they can taste bitter but not as keenly as the supertasters. Because they can taste some bitter, they are usually categorized together with supertasters in many studies. Last, there are AVI/AVI, or nontasters, who are insensitive to bitter. To these nontasters, a PROP-saturated litmus paper tastes like paper. The Monell study found that supertasters (PAV/PAV) rated the glucosinolate vegetables 60 percent more bitter than did nontaster subjects with the AVI/AVI form. Medium tasters fell somewhere in the middle. Surprisingly, supertasters, medium tasters, and nontasters rated other vegetables not containing glucosinolates (such as endive, eggplant, and spinach) equally bitter. How does this relate to the choices in food that we make? The ability to taste—or not taste—various types of bitter or sour compounds likely does lead to differences in diet among people. It is possible that individuals who are genetically more sensitive to some types of bitter would rarely choose foods like broccoli.

To test this idea, Tepper determined tasters and nontasters in a group of 65 preschool children.[16] Next, she gave them five different types of vegetables, both bitter (black olives, cucumbers, and raw broccoli) and nonbitter types (red peppers and carrots), and let them take as much as they wanted. Tepper found that nontaster children ate more bitter vegetables than taster children; the total vegetable consumption was also higher, with nontaster children eating about one serving of vegetables while tasters consumed about one half that amount. Additionally, only 8 percent of the nontaster children refused to eat any vegetables during the free choice in comparison with 32 percent of the taster children. From these results, one can see that being a bitter taster can most certainly influence the food choices one makes.

On the bright side, we know that the more that one is exposed to certain foods, the more likely a preference will be developed for it. Research has found that roughly 70 percent of Caucasians in North America are bitter tasters and 30 percent are nontasters, so it is important to keep exposing one's children to healthy foods so that a preference for these foods will develop over time.[17] Research studies indicate that 5 to 10 exposures may be necessary before a child accepts and/or consumes a new food item.[18] Parents need to be good role models by cooking and eating a wide variety of vegetables (which tend to have more bitter flavors) and offering these taste experiences to their children.

Interestingly, ethnic groups such as the Japanese, Chinese, and West Africans have much smaller numbers of nontasters with as low as 3 percent in some populations with the remaining 97 percent as bitter tasters.[19] The largest group of nontasters resides in India, where taste blindness is found in more than 40 percent of the population. Scientists are unsure as to why some individuals are bitter tasters, but surmise that bitter taste evolved as a defense mechanism to detect potentially harmful toxins.

Understanding Nontasters vs. Tasters

Another difference between tasters and nontasters is that tasters or supertasters have a greater density of tongue papillae than nontasters. Each papillae or tiny bump on the tongue houses several taste buds. Researchers hypothesize this may be one reason why supertasters and tasters perceive a greater intensity of a whole range of tastes including spicy, sweet, and salty stimuli than nontasters. Supertasters' perception of fat content is even enhanced in comparison to nontasters. Supertasters versus medium and nontasters could distinguish differences in fat content in salad dressing composed of either 10 percent or 40 percent fat, whereas nontasters could not.

How exactly does being a supertaster or a taster affect one's food choices? A 2005 Monell Chemical Senses Center study found that both supertaster and taster children preferred higher concentrations of sugary drinks and cereal compared to nontasters.[16] Interestingly, these preferences did not occur in the adult participants, thus the researchers assume that factors other than taste, such as culture and experience, played a role in food preference. Research has found that nontasters seem to desire more of every type of taste: bitter, sweet, spicy, and especially fat.[17] The Monell Chemical Senses Center study also found that supertasters tend to avoid very sweet, high-fat foods as well as bitter foods and typically eat less food in general.[18] Additionally, nontasters prefer higher-fat meats, cheese, and milk more than tasters do.[19] Tepper measured BMI in a small study of 40 middle-aged women and found supertasters were 20 percent thinner than their nontaster counterparts, with a BMI of 23 versus a BMI of 30.[20]

Genes and Taste Discrimination

Genes have been linked to a whole host of eating behaviors in addition to taste discrimination. Several family and twin-based studies have linked one's preference for specific macronutrients such as fat, as well as proteins and carbohydrates, to our genetic makeup. Researchers at Tufts University Human Nutrition Research Center believe they may have pinpointed one of the many genes responsible, a protein called apolipoprotein A-II (APOA2).[21] Through studies, they have shown that this gene is responsible for food preference as well as satiety signals.

Another fascinating eating behavior that researchers are focusing on is the genetic influence on cognitive restraint and disinhibition and susceptibility to hunger. Many studies have linked obesity to disinhibition. Heritability studies have found that heritability based on family and twin studies can be as high as 28 percent for cognitive restraint, 40 percent for disinhibition, and 23 percent for hunger. Studies of genetic influence on macronutrient intake, caloric intake, and meal size show ranges from 20 percent to 40 percent. [22]

APPLYING KNOWLEDGE OF BIOPSYCHOLOGY TO NUTRITION ADHERENCE

Now that we are familiar with some of the biological factors influencing our eating behavior, it is important to utilize this information to our healthy eating advantage. As we know, some of us may have a genetic predisposition to having less dopamine receptors in our brains, leading us not to sense satiety signals as strongly as others. With this knowledge in hand, two psychological strategies can be applied so that one is more sensitive to these signals. Before discussing these strategies, you need to become familiar with the structure of the stomach cavity and how satiety signals are sent to the brain.

Becoming More Sensitive to Our Satiety Signals

Your stomach is a hollow, muscular sac and it is located in the upper left corner of your abdomen, under your rib cage. The average adult stomach is about 10 inches long and can expand to hold about 1 liter to a gallon of food and liquid. When your stomach is empty, its tissues fold in on themselves, somewhat like a deflated balloon. When your stomach fills and expands, the folds slowly disappear. Psychologists have researched the causes of the feeling of hunger and what makes us feel full or satiety.

Our body has several ways to determine how much we should eat. The first method is through our blood sugar level. If your blood sugar level is low, that is a factor that will lead to hunger. After eating, when your blood sugar level rises to normal (or above normal), you will no longer feel hungry. An additional way that our stomach tells us that it is full is the slight stretching of our stomach. Our stomach is a bit stretchy, so when it is full, it takes up a little more room than when it is empty. There are stretch receptors, little nerves, around the stomach that signal the brain when you are full. The last method that our stomach uses to signal us that it is full involves the use of hormones. There are several hormones that travel between our gastrointestinal tract and our central nervous system when we start digesting to alert our brain that we are full. You may not realize that it takes about 15 to 20 minutes after you start eating for the release of the "all-full" hormones and a subsequent rise in the blood sugar level. Because of this "delay," a good rule of thumb is to not eat quickly because you can consume a tremendous amount of food in a short time period and these chemical messengers will not have been even activated. Optimally, you should try to make each meal stretch out to 15 minutes so that your body will be accurately gauging your true level of fullness or satiety. In other words, eat slowly! If you are a fast eater, set a kitchen timer for 15 minutes. Purposely slow down your rate of eating so you take the last bite of food as the timer is beeping. You can do this by engaging in more conversation, setting your utensil down between bites, or taking a sip of water between bites. Regularly practicing these techniques will help you develop a habit of eating more slowly.

Next, let's look at the blood sugar indicator of fullness. Given the choice between breaking down carbohydrates or fats first, your stomach usually chooses the carbohydrates first to serve as an energy source and stores the fat to break down later. The carbohydrates that are converted to energy or sugar ultimately raise your blood sugar level a lot quicker than fats or proteins, alerting your brain that you are full. In summary, you can eat a tremendous amount of fats before feeling full, whereas you can eat a small portion of carbohydrates and achieve satiety much quicker.

Foods High in Satiety

Now let's turn to the second way that your stomach alerts your brain that you are full—the stretch receptors. Optimally what you want to do is to activate your stretch receptors without eating too much food. You want to consume bulky, high-fibrous food that take up a great deal of space in your stomach and activate those stretch receptors to relay the all-full signal to your brain. One way you can bulk up the stomach without eating food is to drink a full glass of water before you sit down and begin to eat. There is no way for your stomach to compress it or break it down and it is calorie free.

In addition to water, what other foods are high in satiety? A head researcher at the University of Sydney, Dr. Susanne Holt and her associates developed a satiety index, which is a listing of foods rated according to their bulk and their ability to make people feel full quicker.[23] Dr. Holt and her colleagues developed this index by having students come in the morning to the lab and eat 240-calorie portions of a specific food. They then rated their feelings of hunger every 15 minutes. During the next 2 hours, students could go to a buffet table and eat as much as they liked, all under the observation of researchers. Using white bread as the baseline of 100, Dr. Holt and her team of researchers scored 38 different foods that were given to the students. Foods scoring higher than 100 were judged to be a certain percentage more satisfying than white bread, while those under 100 were a particular percentage less satisfying. Foods that have a higher satiety index keep hunger down longer and would be better choices for those who want to lose weight.

An interesting finding from Dr. Holt's study is that some foods such as croissants are only half as satisfying as white bread, while potatoes are more than three times as satisfying, but french fries did not score well! As a group, fruits ranked at the top for foods to choose with a satiety index 1.7 times higher than white bread. Some of the high-satiety foods listed in **Table 11–1** (such as popcorn) should be used only as snacking foods because many of

The Satiety Index

Note: All food are compared to white bread, ranked as "100%." Each food is rated by the extent that it satisfied the participants' hunger.

Tip: If you want to lose weight, **stay away** from the LOWER numbers!

Bakery Products		Carbohydrate-Rich Foods	
Croissant	47%	White bread	100%
Cake	65%	French fries	116%
Doughnuts	68%	White pasta	119%
Cookies	120%	Brown rice	132%
Crackers	127%	White rice	138%
Snacks and Confectionary		Grain bread	154%
Mars candy bar	70%	Whole-meal bread	157%
Peanuts	84%	Brown pasta	188%
Yogurt	88%	Potatoes	323%
Crisps	91%	**Protein-Rich Foods**	
Ice cream	96%	Lentils	133%
Jellybeans	118%	Cheese	146%
Popcorn	154%	Eggs	150%
Breakfast Cereals		Baked beans	168%
Muesli	100%	Beef	176%
Sustain	112%	Fish	225%
Special K	116%	**Fruits**	
Cornflakes	118%	Bananas	118%
Honey Smacks	132%	Grapes	162%
All-Bran	151%	Apples	197%
Porridge/Oatmeal	209%	Oranges	202%

Table 11–1 The Satiety Index.

Source: Adapted from Holt, S.H., Miller, J.C., Petocz, P. and Farmakalidis, E. (1995). A satiety index of common foods. *European Journal Clinical Nutrition, 49(9)*: 675–90.

these foods lack the nutrients that our bodies need on a daily basis. Ultimately when we reach for a snack, we should be thinking bulk and high satiety.

Visualizing Satiety

In addition to consuming bulky foods to intensify one's feelings of satiety, one can also use the process of visualization. Focus on the concept of gastric bypass surgery for a minute. In normal digestion, food passes through the stomach and enters the small intestine where most of the nutrients and calories are absorbed. Food then passes into the large intestine (colon), and the remaining waste is eventually excreted. Gastric bypass surgery makes the stomach smaller by creating a small pouch at the top of the stomach with surgical staples. This small pouch, which is capable of only holding 2 to 3 ounces of volume, is then connected directly to the middle portion of the small intestine and bypasses the rest of the larger original stomach and part of the small intestine. This procedure allows the person to feel full more quickly than when the stomach was its original size. This, in turn, reduces the amount of food eaten, leading to a severe reduction in total daily calories consumed, and initiates weight loss. Food also bypasses part of the small intestine causing less calories to be absorbed. After the surgery, the recovery time is usually 3–5 weeks and the patient will typically lose about one-third of his or her weight.

Why not apply the process of visualization to your stomach in the form of a mental gastric bypass to intensify one's satiety signals? Try visualizing your stomach not at the full 10 inches that it is and able to hold a gallon of food and water, but as a mere, let's say, 5-by-5 inch receptacle or about a 1- to 1 1/2-cup capacity (this is all visualization so you can choose the new measurement of your stomach).

Visualization is the use of a positive suggestion through mental imagery to change a mental and/or physiological state. When you create a mental picture, your body can actually respond to the visualization as if it were a real experience. It is a powerful tool you can use to gain control of your mind, emotions, and body. It can also help to bring about desired changes in your behavior because your subconscious tries to make your behavior consistent with your mental images and thoughts.

Visualization has been successfully used in many life venues. Sports psychologists rely heavily on the process of visualization when coaching their clients. A prominent documented example of the effectiveness of visualization occurred with the 1976 U.S. Olympic ski team, The psychologist working with the team had the team members visualize, not the winning of a gold medal, but on the "means" by which they were to do it. More specifically, the skiers visualized themselves careening through the entire course, experiencing each bump and turn in their minds. The team was not expected to do well in the Olympics, but had great success that year. Visualization is now a standard tool in training Olympic athletes.

Throughout each day and especially during meal time, visualize your stomach cavity as only able to hold a fist full or about 1 cup of food at its fullest capacity. The more often you engage in this process of visualization, the more your brain can help keep your eating behavior consistent with your mental image.

Counseling Techniques

For healthcare advisors, knowing that people are predisposed to a certain behavior can help direct the development of their counseling strategies. Let's consider an individual's differences in taste perception. Nontasters generally want flavor and fat, which makes following a reduced calorie diet extremely difficult for them. Supertasters, in comparison, tend to avoid strong flavors and healthy vegetables because most vegetables taste bitter. Healthcare advisors should suggest that their nontaster clients enhance the foods on their eating plan with healthy spices or sweet condiments. Spices, herbs, and seasoning mixes can kick up the flavor to their liking. Examples of flavorful fresh herbs are basil, thyme, oregano, and cilantro. Sodium-free seasoning mixtures of dried herbs are also available at the grocery store. Condiments such as sweet pickle relish, Dijon mustard, salsa, hot sauce, and others can also add significant flavor with very minimal calories. The advisor can sit down with his or her client and devise a list of the flavor enhancers that the client would be willing to try.

For supertasters, the advisor should recommend lightly steamed raw vegetables or adding a healthy condiment of their choosing to decrease bitterness. Again a list of condiments from which the client could draw from would be optimal.

As one can see having a genetic predisposition that affects one's eating behavior does not mean one is doomed to maladaptive eating behaviors. Simply being aware of one's predispositions is half the battle.

You Diagnose It

ADHERENCE SCENARIO 1

Amelia and her mother have always had a strong fondness for anything sweet. Amelia has noticed that there seems to be several days during each month in which she craves sweets and feels like she has no control over her eating behavior.

1. As a healthcare advisor, give Amelia a biological explanation for her eating behavior.
2. Develop a game plan so that Amelia can preplan for these biologically motivated cravings.

ADHERENCE SCENARIO 2

Mike's brother and both of his parents are obese. Mike has relayed to his registered dietician that once he starts eating, he is unable to stop until his stomach feels sick.

1. As a healthcare advisor, give Mike a biological explanation for his eating behavior.
2. Develop a game plan so that Mike is able to recognize the signs that his body is full and inhibit his eating behavior.

Review

✓ The application of the principles of biology to the study of mental processes and behavior is referred to as biopsychology or neuropsychology.

✓ One of the earliest techniques to study the relationship between brain regions and resulting behavior that researchers used was studying brain-damaged individuals.

✓ Another method that biopsychologists rely on to understand the relationship between brain and behavior is through creating lesions. A lesion is a brain region of interest that is destroyed or stimulated so that changes such as diminished or enhanced performance on some behavioral measure can be observed.

✓ To measure the neural activity of that region or of a specific neuron(s), the researcher will attach electrodes to the scalp of the subject to recode the firing activity of the neurons. Functional magnetic resonance imaging (fMRI) is another method to measure enhanced neural activity by recording the cerebral blood flow, which indicates activity of larger portions of the brain. These changes in blood flow can be detected in an MRI apparatus.

✓ Research by Amico and Vollmer has found that animals deficient in the hormone oxytocin are more likely to develop a sweet tooth.

✓ Slight changes in TSH, the thyroid stimulating hormone produced in the thyroid gland located in the lower front of the neck, have been shown to affect weight gain and loss.

✓ Neurotransmitters, which are chemicals that relay, amplify, and modulate signals between a neuron and another cell, have been found to affect eating behavior. The new field of nutrigenetics studies the genetic influences on what we eat, as well as how much we eat and even our eating behavior. Nutrigenomics is another buzzword in the field and refers to the influence of diet on genes, mainly related to health and disease states such as obesity, cancer, and heart disease.

✓ Genes have been linked to a whole host of eating behaviors in addition to taste discrimination. Several family and twin-based studies have linked one's preference for specific macronutrients such as fat, as well as proteins and carbohydrates, to our genetic makeup.

✓ A researcher at the University of Sydney, Dr. Susanne Holt and her colleagues developed a satiety index, which is a listing of foods based on their bulkiness and their ability to make people feel full quicker.

D.I.E.T. (Do I Eat This?)

TIPS TO CONSIDER WHEN REACHING FOR A PIECE OF FOOD

- Am I eating because of a hormonal influence?
- Am I missing my body's signals of satiety?
- Am I avoiding healthy foods just because they are bitter tasting to me?
- Should I be consuming a bulky food that increases my satiety level instead?

REFERENCES

1. Stice, E., Spoor, S., Bohon, C., & Small, D. (2008). Relation between obesity and blunted striatal response to food is moderated by the TaqIA1 gene. *Science, 322*, 449–452.
2. Brater, D.C., & Daly, W.J. (2000). Clinical pharmacology in the Middle Ages: Principles that presage the 21st century, *Clinical Pharmacology & Therapeutics, 67*(5), 447–450.
3. James, W. (1981). *The Principles of Psychology*, Cambridge, MA: Harvard University Press. Originally published in 1890.
4. Harlow, J.M. (1868). Recovery from the passage of an iron through the head. *Publications of the Massachusetts Medical Society, 2*, 327–347.
5. Harlow, J.M. (1869). *Recovery from the Passage of an Iron Bar Through the Head.* Boston: Clapp.
6. Wang, G.J., Tomasi, D., Backus, W., Wang, R., Telang, F., Geliebter, A., et al. (2008). Gastric distention activates satiety circuitry in the human brain. *Neuroimage, 39*(4), 1824–1831.

7. Wang, G.J., Volkow, N.D., Telang F., Jayne, M., Ma, Y., Pradhan, K., et al. (2009). Evidence of gender differences in the ability to inhibit brain activation elicited by food stimulation. *Proceedings of the National Academy of Sciences, 106*(4), 1249–1254.

8. Ibid.

9. Farooqi, S., Bullmore, E., Keogh, J., Gillard, J., O'Rahilly, S., & Fletcher, P.C. (2007). Leptin regulates striatal regions and human eating behavior. *Science, 317*, 1355.

10. Amico, J.A., Morris, M., & Vollmer, R.R. (2001). Mice deficient in oxytocin manifest increases in saline consumption following overnight water deprivation. *American Journal of Physiology Regulatory, Integrative, Comparative Physiology, 281*, R1368–R1373.

11. Fox, C.S., Weiss, R.E., & Brown, R.L. (2008). Relations of thyroid function to body weight: Cross-sectional and longitudinal observations in a community-based sample. *Archives of Internal Medicine, 168*, 587–592.

12. Kaye, W.H., Frank, G.K., Bailer, U.F., & Henry, S.E. (2005). Neurobiology of anorexia nervosa: Clinical implications of alterations of the function of serotonin and other neuronal systems. *International Journal of Eating Disorders, 37*, S20-S21.

13. Kaye, W.H., Bailer, U.F., Frank G.K., Wagner, A., Hentry S.E. (2005). Brain imaging of serotonin after recovery from anorexia and bulimia nervosa. *Physiology & Behavior, 86*(1-2), 15-7.

14. Nabhan, G.P. (2004). *Why Some Like It Hot: Food, Genes, and Cultural Diversity.* Washington, DC: Island Press.

15. Mennella, J.A., Pepino, M.Y., & Reed, D.R. (2005). Genetic and environmental determinants of bitter and sweet preferences. *Pediatrics, 115*(2), e216–e222.

16. Tepper, B.J. (2006). PROP sensitivity and food selection in children. *Network Health Dietitian*, 10–11.

17. Nabhan, G.P. (2004). *Why Some Like It Hot: Food, Genes, and Cultural Diversity.* Washington, DC: Island Press.

18. Mennella, J.A., Pepino, M.Y., & Reed, D.R. (2005). Genetic and environmental determinants of bitter and sweet preferences. *Pediatrics, 115*(2), e216–e222.

19. Nabhan, G.P. (2004). *Why Some Like It Hot: Food, Genes, and Cultural Diversity.* Washington, DC: Island Press.

20. Tepper, B. J., & Ullrich, N. V. (2002). Influence of genetic taste sensitivity to 6-npropylthiouracil (PROP), dietary restraint, and disinhibition on body mass index in middle-aged women. *Physiology and Behavior, 75*(3), 305–312.

21. Genetics linked to diet patterns and fat fondness. (2007). *Tufts University Health & Nutrition Letter, 25*(7), 1–2.

22. Rankinen, T., Bouchard, C. (2006). Genetics of food intake and eating behavior phenotypes in humans. *Annual Review of Nutrition.* (26): 413–434.

23. Holt, S.H., Miller, J.C., Petocz, P., & Farmakalidis, E. (1995). A satiety index of common foods. *European Journal Clinical Nutrition, 49*(9), 675–690.

Chapter 12

Sleep, Water Intake, and Eating Behavior

LEARNING OBJECTIVES

By the end of this chapter, the reader will be able to:

1. Understand the value of examining eating behavior as it relates to the biological processes of sleep and water intake.
2. Become familiar with the relationship between sleep deprivation and appetite stimulation.
3. Become aware of the association between water intake, eating behavior, and the body's metabolism.
4. Apply psychological strategies to obtain the optimal amount of sleep and water intake so that adhering to a healthy eating plan is facilitated.

Dinner at the Vending Machine?

THE GRAVEYARD SHIFT AND OBESITY

Over three million Americans work the graveyard or night shift, which is about 3.5 percent of the total work force.[1] Adjusting to a nighttime work schedule is very difficult because it works against the body's natural daily rhythms (as well as society's rhythms) for such endeavors as eating and family events.

However, it is possible to adapt to a night work schedule as graveyard workers attest; some workers even grow to relish it. Despite its adaptability, there are major health hazards of working the night shift. The obvious hazard is sleep deprivation. Without quality sleep, the brain and organs do not have the opportunity to restore themselves. Over time, sleep deprivation increases the risk for high blood pressure and stroke. Also, the hormones responsible for keeping the employee alert and able to handle the problems they encounter on the job do not naturally shift to night time and unusual hours.

But of particular importance to this textbook, the incidence of obesity is significantly high among graveyard workers, which increases their risk for diabetes.[2] Why obesity? The irregular sleep and eating patterns of working at night disrupt normal digestive patterns, which adhere to a circadian rhythm of the physiological changes in a 24-hour day. Additionally, these irregular hours also cause upset stomachs, ulcers, and constipation. The rate of stress-related gastrointestinal disorders is up to 150 percent higher among workers who work the night shift.[3] These individuals are far less likely to eat a nutritious diet, in part, because they are not home during regular family meals and cafeterias and restaurants are more likely closed. Thus, one of the prominent sources for food turns out to be vending machines that contain fatty foods. Many workers eagerly take on these irregular shifts, but need to be alerted to the potential life-threatening hazards that come with the job.

THE BASICS ABOUT SLEEP

This final chapter covers the most crucial biological processes that have the greatest impact on eating adherence behavior: sleep and water intake. By understanding these biological processes in greater detail as well as their effect on eating behavior, you will see the need to implement psychological strategies to ensure that a reasonable number of hours of sleep and the recommended amount of water are attained on a daily basis.

Sleep Defined

Sleep is the regular cycle of rest that occurs in all mammals, birds, and fish. When an individual is in a state of sleep, that person is actually not unconscious, but is in a natural state of rest characterized by a reduction in voluntary body movement and decreased awareness of their surroundings. Sleep is induced by our body's natural daily circadian rhythms, and by hormonal and environmental factors, too. Sleep is believed to perform a restorative function for the body and brain.[4]

Studying the Process of Sleep

Because of today's ever-increasing technology and advances in the fields of neurology, neuroscience, and genetics, scientists are able to study sleep patterns in depth. One way that scientists study sleep patterns is by recording the electrical impulses generated by the brain by using a device called an electroencephalograph (EEG). The cycle of sleep and wakefulness is controlled by the brain stem, external stimuli, and several types of hormones produced by the hypothalamus. The neurohormone, melatonin, has been found to be at its highest level during the night and promotes sleep. Adenosine, a nucleoside that is involved in producing energy for biochemical processes, slowly accumulates in the human brain during wakefulness, but decreases during sleep; scientists theorize that its accumulation during the day encourages sleep. The stimulant properties of caffeinated substances are attributed to negating the effects of adenosine.

The suprachiasmatic nucleus (SCN), located in the brain's hypothalamus plays a prominent role in the regulation of circadian rhythms. The SCN is influenced by external light and also develops its own rhythm in isolation. When it encounters light, it sends messages to the pineal gland that signal it to cease secreting melatonin.

According to EEG recordings of human sleep patterns, five stages of sleep occur. Stage 1, which is called nonrapid eye movement (non-REM or NREM) sleep, accounts for 75 to 80 percent of total sleep time. This stage is also referred to as "drowsy sleep" in which the subject loses muscle tone and conscious awareness of the external surroundings.[5]

Next, stage 2 is characterized by "sleep spindles" seen in the EEG; in which conscious awareness of the environment lowers even more. This stage accounts for 45 to 55 percent of one's total sleep cycle. Stage 3, with its delta waves, functions primarily as a transition into stage 4 and accounts for 3 to 8 percent of total sleep time. Stage 4 is characterized by true delta sleep, the slowest brain waves. It dominates the first third of the night and accounts for 10 to 15 percent of total sleep time. Stage 4 is believed to be the deepest stage of sleep because it is extremely difficult to wake a subject in this state. Interestingly, this is the stage in which night terrors and sleepwalking can occur. Stage 5, REM sleep, is connected with dreaming. The EEG in this period is aroused and resembles stage 1, and sometimes includes beta waves.

Sleep progresses in cycles of NREM and REM phases. In humans, the cycle of REM and NREM is about 90 minutes. Each stage of sleep has a specific physiological function. For example, during stages 3 and 4, growth occurs, levels of hormones increase, and changes in immune function occur. The wide variety of illnesses associated with sleep deprivation account for its restorative function. NREM sleep has been found to be an anabolic state characterized by physiological processes of growth and rejuvenation of the organism's immune, nervous, muscular, and skeletal systems. Sleep also restores neurons and increases production of brain proteins and certain hormones.

Wakefulness may perhaps be viewed as a cyclical, temporary, hyperactive catabolic state during which the organism acquires nourishment and procreates.

A typical misnomer is that every person needs 8 hours of sleep. The amount of sleep needed is different for every person and is individually and biologically determined. However, as a rule of thumb, 8 hours of sleep is suggested. Interestingly, sleep scientists tell us that you cannot "store up" on your sleep by sleeping more on the weekends in preparation for the normal work week. Another commonly held view is that the amount of sleep one requires decreases as one ages, but this is not generally the case.

SLEEP DEPRIVATION AND HUNGER

Now that we are familiar with the basics about sleep, let's delve into how sleep deprivation is associated with hunger and ultimately, obesity. Scientists have found that sleep deprivation increases levels of a hunger hormone and decreases levels of a hormone that makes you feel full. This process may lead to overeating and weight gain and would explain why so many Americans who are chronically sleep deprived are also overweight. It also makes sense that new parents and shift workers who are sleep deprived gain a great deal of weight. Scientists believe that getting enough sleep is a critical aspect of weight management.

Sixty-five percent of Americans are overweight, which increases their risk of heart disease, type 2 diabetes, cancer, and other diseases. This percentage is especially significant when compared to the fact that an estimated 63 percent of U.S. adults do not get the suggested 8 hours of sleep a night, according to the National Sleep Foundation.[6] This research also indicates that the average adult gets 6.9 hours of sleep on weeknights and 7.5 hours on weekends, for a daily average of 7 hours.

Dr. Eve Van Cauter, the director of the Research Laboratory on Sleep, Chronobiology, and Neuroendocrinology at the University of Chicago School of Medicine, extensively investigated the association between sleep deprivation and appetite stimulation.[7] In her study with her colleagues, she examined 12 normal-weight, 22-year-old men who came to a hospital laboratory to sleep and eat dinner and breakfast. On one occasion, the participants were limited to 4 hours in bed for each of two consecutive nights. At another time, they were allowed up to 10 hours in bed for two nights. The participants' blood was drawn at regular intervals, and they were asked questions regarding their hunger. Van Cauter's research revealed that sleep deprivation activates a small part of the hypothalamus, the region of the brain that is also involved in appetite regulation. Van Cauter looked at two critical hormones in particular, both involved in regulating food intake: ghrelin and leptin.

Ghrelin is an appetite-stimulating hormone released generally by the stomach. When ghrelin levels are high, people feel hungry. In comparison, leptin, considered a satiety or fullness hormone, is released by the fat cells and signals the brain with regard to the current energy balance of the body. When leptin levels are high, a signal is sent to the brain that the body has enough food, and the person feels full while low levels of leptin indicate starvation and increase appetite. The hormones "have been called the yin and yang of hunger," Van Cauter says. "One is the accelerator for eating (ghrelin), and the other is the brake (leptin)."[8] More specifically, Van Cauter found in this study:

- Leptin levels were 18 percent lower and ghrelin levels were 28 percent higher after the participants slept for 4 hours.
- The sleep-deprived participants who had the biggest hormonal changes also said they felt the most hunger and craved. carbohydrate-rich foods, such as cakes, candy, ice cream, and bread. Those participants who had the smallest hormonal changes reported being the least hungry.

Sleep scientists at the University of Wisconsin and Stanford University (Mignot et al. 2009) found similar findings with their study that tracked 1,024 people ages 30 to 60.[9] Participants from the Wisconsin Sleep Cohort Study took sleep tests and blood tests every 4 years and discussed their sleep habits. The specific findings from this study were the following:

- Participants who typically slept 5 hours a night had a 14.9 percent higher level of ghrelin and a 15.5 percent lower level of leptin than those participants who slept 8 hours.
- Those participants who normally slept less than 7.7 hours had a slightly higher BMI.

Similarly, a study conducted at Columbia University in New York used government data on 6,115 people to compare sleep patterns and obesity. The researchers found that people who sleep 2 to 4 hours a night are 73 percent more likely to be obese than those who get 7 to 9 hours. Those participants who get 5 or more hours of sleep a night were 50 percent more likely to be obese than normal sleepers. Those participants who sleep 6 hours were 23 percent more likely to be obese. Finally, those participants who get 10 or more hours are 11 percent less likely to be obese. What is interesting about these findings is that we used to think that sleep-deprived individuals used food as a pick-me-up when they were tired, but the data now indicate that these individuals are indeed truly hungry due to a hormonal state.[10]

APPLYING PSYCHOLOGY TO FACILITATE ADEQUATE SLEEP

With the understanding of the crucial link between lack of sleep and hunger, we can see how difficult it would be in a sleep-deprived state to adhere to one's eating plan. Thankfully, there are many approaches and psychological strategies that are available to improve falling asleep and staying asleep. Here are several strategies that a person can utilize:

1. Decrease the light level in your sleeping environment. Studies have shown that the brain has a separate neural pathway to the optical nerve, separate from the visual path, to detect whether it's day or night. This detection system could have a direct effect on sleep inducement.

2. Classically condition your body to feel drowsy. Develop a bedtime routine 30 minutes prior to the time that you would like to sleep. This routine should be calm and quiet, so as to slow down your metabolic rate. This quiet time should not consist of any stimulating activities such as using the computer, watching television, playing video games, doing office work, or housework. However, reading or other light mental activity should be fine. Try to ensure that the 30-minute routine is the same each night so that the routine conditions your body to become drowsy.

3. Ensure that your sleeping position is comfortable and gives enough support, particularly for the lower back area.

4. Listen to quiet, slow-paced music to facilitate sleep inducement.

5. Do not use your bed for other activities (e.g., watching TV, doing homework, working on one's laptop) so that the body and mind will maintain an association between getting into bed and sleeping.

6. Avoid drinking beverages containing caffeine prior to bedtime (e.g., coffee, tea, soft drinks, energy drinks).

7. Studies have shown sleep inducement is increased when body temperature is lowered.[11] Crack open a window or turn on a fan to cool down your sleeping environment.

8. Try to avoid eating a large evening meal within 4 hours of bedtime. Large meals may lead to abdominal discomfort or heartburn which might interrupt sleep.

9. Try not to engage in vigorous physical activity right before going to bed because your heart rate will be high.

WATER INTAKE AND METABOLISM

The second biological process that is an extremely crucial factor in any eating plan is water intake. Water is your body's primary chemical component and makes up, on average, 60 percent of your body weight. Every system in your body is dependent on water to function. For instance, water flushes toxins out of vital organs, carries nutrients to your cells, and gives a moist environment for ear, nose, and throat tissues. A lack of water in the body can lead to dehydration, a state that occurs when you don't have enough water in your body to carry out normal functions. Mild dehydration can even drain your energy and make you feel tired. Physical symptoms of mild dehydration or a fluid loss equal to less than 5 percent of body weight include thirst, dry skin, dry mouth and throat, rapid pulse, weakness, reduced quantity of urine, decreased mental and muscle function, and fainting. Symptoms of fluid loss greater than 5 percent of body weight include pale skin, bluish tint to lips and fingertips, confused state, rapid and shallow breathing, and a weak irregular pulse. If immediate medical attention is not sought, coma and death are a strong possibility.

Each day, we lose water through breathing, perspiration, urine, and bowel movements. To make your body function properly, you need to replenish its water supply by consuming beverages and foods that contain water. Many theories have set out to determine approximate water needs for the average, healthy adult who lives in a temperate climate.

Theories of Water Intake

One theory is termed the replacement approach. We know that the average urine output for adults is about 1.5 liters (6.3 cups) per day.[12] Additionally, we lose close to an additional liter of water per day by breathing, sweating, and bowel movements. Food typically accounts for 20 percent of your total fluid intake, so if you imbibe 2 liters of water or another type of beverage a day (a little more than 8 cups) in addition to your normal diet, you will generally replace the lost fluids.

Another theory suggests eight 8-ounce glasses of water a day. This approach to water intake is the "8 × 8 rule" in which you drink eight 8-ounce glasses of water a day (about 1.9 liters). The rule could also be interpreted as "drink eight 8-ounce glasses of fluid a day," because all fluids count toward the daily total. It should be noted that is approach isn't supported by scientific evidence, though many people use this basic rule as a guideline for how much water and other fluids to drink. Keep in mind that you may need to modify your total fluid intake depending on how active you are, the climate you live in, your health status, and if you're pregnant or breastfeeding.

As a general guideline, the Dietary Reference Intake or DRI recommendation (a set of nutritional standards developed by a committee of nutrition experts) is 9 cups per day of fluid for adult women and 13 cups of fluid per day for adult men (average environmental temperature and normal diet). This amount of fluid includes not only water but all other beverages a person may consume.

Causes for Fluid Loss

If you exercise or do any activity that makes you sweat, you need to drink extra water to compensate for the fluid loss. An extra 400 to 600 milliliters (about 1.5 to 2.5 cups) of water should be adequate for short periods of exercise. However, for intense exercise lasting more than an hour, fluids containing electrolytes (such as sports drinks) are recommended. The additional amount of fluid is dependent on how much you sweat during exercise, the duration of your exercise, and the form of exercise that you are doing. Athletes can calculate out their individual fluid needs by taking their body weight before an event and after an event. For example, if an athlete weighs 165 pounds prior to an event, drinks 14 ounces during the event, and then weighs 163 after the event, he has lost 2 pounds or 32 ounces of fluid. To better match his fluid intake with his bodies fluid needs, the next time he participates in the same event, given that the conditions are similar (i.e., the outdoor temperature and humidity level is the same), he should drink 46 ounces of fluid during the event to prevent fluid loss (14 ounces + an additional 32 ounces = 46 ounces).

The environment that one is in, whether it is hot or humid, can make you sweat and requires additional intake of fluid. Also, keep in mind that heated indoor air also can cause your skin to lose moisture during the winter months. High altitudes (greater than 8,200 feet) may also trigger increased urination and more rapid breathing, which use up more of your fluid that is on hand.

Illness is another factor to be aware of because fever, vomiting, and diarrhea cause your body to lose additional fluids. In these instances, one should drink more water or oral rehydration solutions, like sport drinks. Further, you may need increased fluid intake if conditions such as a bladder infection or urinary tract stones develop.

Foods for Hydration

Although it's a great idea to keep water within reach at all times, you don't need to rely only on what you drink to satisfy your fluid needs. What you eat also provides a significant portion of your fluid needs. On average, food provides about 20 percent of total water intake, while the remaining 80 percent comes from water and beverages of all kinds. For example, many fruits and vegetables, such as watermelon and tomatoes, are 90 percent to 100 percent water by weight. Drinks such as milk and juice also are comprised primarily of water. Additionally, beer, wine, and caffeinated drinks can contribute, but these should not be a predominant portion of your daily total fluid consumption. Remember that water is the optimal fluid because it's calorie free and very inexpensive.

Too Much Water?

Can we drink too much water? Water is necessary and most people don't drink enough but drinking excessive volumes of water over a short period of time can be dangerous and life threatening. *Hyponatremia* is a medical condition that occurs when the sodium level of the bloodstream drops to a dangerously low level, low enough to stop the heart and cause heart failure and death. This can be caused by profuse sweating with a significant loss of sodium (heavy sweating for 3 hours or more) or by drinking too much water and diluting the sodium level in the bloodstream. It is a rare occurrence, however, each year, there is usually one story in the media about an inexperienced marathon runner who during their race, overhydrates, develops hyponatremia, and dies.

Confusing Thirst for Hunger

According to the *American Dietetic Association Complete Food and Nutrition Guide,* thirst can be commonly mistaken for hunger, even though the body senses these states through separate mechanisms.[13] Our hunger sensors detect changes in one's energy fuel supply (glucose, sugar levels) as a signal of hunger, whereas, our thirst sensors detect increases in one's blood levels of sodium or decreases in blood volume as a signal of thirst. One explanation for misinterpretation of signals is that eating can bring a sense of solace to thirst because some foods do have water contained within them. A second reason is that both thirst and hunger cravings usually come at the same time: during meal times. Another reason that we confuse thirst for hunger is that with dehydration comes a feeling of fatigue. Many times we interpret this feeling of lethargy as being due to a lack of energy fuel (sugar) and this produces a false sense of hunger. Then, if we do "mistakenly" consume food, our body needs additional water to manufacture digestive juices to digest the food. This produces a vicious cycle due to a misinterpretation of thirst signals for hunger. As one can imagine, consistently misinterpreting thirst signals as hunger can play havoc when trying to adhere to one's eating plan. The American Dietetic Association recommends drinking a glass of water and waiting 10 minutes to see if one is still hungry or if it was thirst that was stimulating one's appetite prior to indulging in a snack or early meal.

APPLYING PSYCHOLOGY TO STAYING HYDRATED

Just like sleep deprivation, a lack of water can stimulate the appetite, making adherence to one's eating plan very difficult. Therefore, it is crucial that one stay adequately hydrated throughout each day. Here are some strategies and psychological approaches to remain hydrated:

1. It is typically not a good idea to use thirst alone as a signal for when to drink. It is possible that by the time you become thirsty, you already may be slightly dehydrated.

2. Additionally, remember that as you get older, your body is less able to detect dehydration and send your brain signals of thirst.

3. Classically condition your body and mind to drink a glass of water with each meal. After several repetitive pairings of eating a meal and drinking water, you should become conditioned to feel thirsty for water upon seeing or even smelling the meal.

4. Hydrate yourself before, during, and after exercise.

5. In Western society, the typical diet is made up of packaged or convenient foods. These foods frequently consist of high levels of salt and salt contains sodium. Therefore, if a diet is primarily comprised of high-sodium foods, then naturally the sodium intake also rises and extra weight is gained quickly because the body holds onto water. The opposite occurs when an individual reduces food intake or the amount of fast food or prepackaged food one eats. One will find that with this change in diet that they will quickly shed several pounds. It is important to remember that a percentage of the loss will be water because the body is no longer in a state of sodium imbalance.

6. Measure out your intended water intake at the beginning of each day. Place the glasses or bottles of water throughout the house or office in areas that you are likely to frequent, just as marketers strategically place products in grocery store aisles. The more that you see the water containers, the more you will be likely to drink them throughout the day. To add to the water's appeal, place it in decorative glasses or add in a cucumber or a sprig of mint for a spa experience.

7. When feeling hungry, drink a glass of water and wait 10 minutes to see if thirst was stimulating your appetite instead of true hunger.

8. Consume foods that contain a larger percentage of water. Some foods that contain a high percentage of water content are found in **Table 12–1**.

Table 12–1 Foods High in Water.

Food	Serving Size	Percent Water
Lettuce	$1^1/_2$ cup	95
Watermelon	$1^1/_2$ cup	92
Broccoli	$1^1/_2$ cup	91
Grapefruit	$1^1/_2$ cup	91
Milk	1 cup	89
Orange Juice	$^3/_4$ cup	88
Carrot	$1^1/_2$ cup	87
Apple	One medium	84

Source: Adapted from Duyff, R.L. (2006). *American Dietetic Association Complete Food and Nutrition Guide.* Hoboken, NJ: Wiley.

You Diagnose It

ADHERENCE SCENARIO 1

Belithia drinks three diet sodas throughout her 8-hour day at work and heats up a prepackaged frozen meal for lunch. However, Belithia still feels hungry every 2 hours and has great difficulty adhering to her eating plan.

1. Give a biological explanation for Belithia's frequent bouts of hunger.

2. Develop a plan so that Belithia can classically condition herself to hydrate herself with each meal.

ADHERENCE SCENARIO 2

Reynaldo is a full-time student at the university and also work 20 hours a week from 5 to 11 PM as a server at a local Italian restaurant. After work, Reynaldo usually takes out his laptop and starts in on his homework on his bed. Typically, Reynaldo finishes his homework around 2 AM and rises at 6 AM to make it to his 7 AM class. After 1 month into the semester, Reynaldo has found that he has gained 8 pounds.

1. Give a biological explanation for Reynaldo's weight gain.

2. Discuss four situational changes that Reynaldo could make to maintain a healthy weight.

Review

✓ Sleep is the regular state of rest seen in all mammals, birds, and fish. When an individual is in a state of sleep, that person is actually not unconscious, but is in a natural state of rest categorized by a reduction in voluntary body movement and decreased awareness of the surroundings.

✓ One way that scientists study sleep patterns is by recording the electrical impulses generated by the brain by using a device called an electroencephalograph (EEG).

✓ We used to think that sleep-deprived individuals used food as a pick-me-up when they were tired, but the data now indicate that these individuals are indeed truly hungry due to a hormonal state.

✓ Water is your body's primary chemical component and makes up, on average, 60 percent of your body weight.

✓ Each day, we lose water through breathing, perspiration, urine, and bowel movements. To make your body function properly, you need to replenish its water supply by consuming beverages and foods that contain water.

✓ Many theories have set out to determine approximate water needs for the average, healthy adult who lives in a temperate climate. One theory is termed the replacement approach; another theory is the eight 8-ounce glasses of water a day approach.

✓ According to the *American Dietetic Association Complete Food and Nutrition Guide*, thirst can be commonly mistaken for hunger, even though the body senses these states through separate mechanisms.

D.I.E.T. (Do I Eat This?)

TIPS TO CONSIDER WHEN REACHING FOR A PIECE OF FOOD

- Is lack of sleep stimulating my appetite?
- Is my thirst actually stimulating my appetite?
- Should I have a glass of water instead?
- Should I have a piece of fruit that contains fluid instead?

REFERENCES

1. U.S. Bureau of Labor Statistics. (2009). American Time Use Survey. Available at: www.bls.gov/tus. Accessed July, 2009.
2. Gomez-Santos, C., Gomez-Abellan, P., Madrid, J., Hernandez-Morante, J., Lujan, J.A., Ordovas, J.M., et al. (2009). Circadian rhythm of clock genes in human adipose explants. *Obesity, 10,* 1000–1038.

3. Ibid.
4. Gottlieb, D.J., Punjabi, N.M., Newman, A.B., Resnick, H.E., Redline, S., & Baldwin, C.M. (2005). Association of sleep time with diabetes mellitus and impaired glucose tolerance. *Archives of Internal Medicine, 165*(8), 863–867.
5. Meddis, R. (1979). The evolution and function of sleep. In D.A. Oakley & H.C. Plotkin (Eds.), *Brain, Behaviour and Evolution*, London, UK: Methuen.
6. National Sleep Foundation. Fact sheet. Available at: www.sleepfoundation.org. Accessed July, 2009
7. Spiegel, K., Tasali, E., Penev, P., & Van Cauter, E. (2004). Brief communication: Sleep curtailment in healthy young men is associated with decreased leptin levels, elevated ghrelin levels, and increased hunger and appetite. *Annals of Internal Medicine, 141*, 846–850.
8. Ibid.
9. Taheri, S., Lin, L., Austin, D., Young, T., Mignot, E., (2004). Short sleep duration is associated with reduced leptin, evaluated ghrelin and increased body mass index. *PloS Medicine, 1*(3), e62.
10. Horne, J. (2008). Short sleep is a questionable risk factor for obesity and related disorders: Statistical vs. clinical significance. *Biological Psychology, 77*(3), 266–276.
11. Franken, T., Tobler, I., & Borbely, A.A. (1992). Cortical temperature and EEG slow-wave activity in the rat: Analysis of vigilance state related changes. *Pfugers Archives, 420*(5–6), 500–507.
12. Mayo Clinic. Water: How much should you drink every day? Available at: www.mayoclinic.com/health/water. Accessed July, 2009.
13. Duyff, R.L. (2006). *American Dietetic Association Complete Food and Nutrition Guide.* Hoboken, NJ: Wiley.

Index